So You Wanna Be A Doctor??
The Untold Stories of Medical, Dental, and Veterinary Residents
by
Shermian P. Daniel, M.D. and Richard S. Daniel

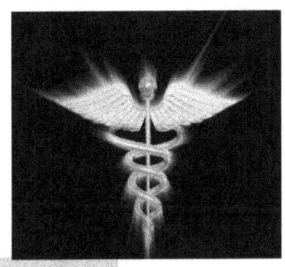

Wagner Wolf, LLC

South Orange   *   Philadelphia

© 2013 Wagner Wolf, LLC

Printed and bound in the United States of America. First Printing: November 2009. Layout consultation provided by Gadfellows LLC. All pictures and cover art provided by Wagner Wolf, LLC and istockphoto.com

ISBN 9781484880180

Library of Congress Control Number: 2009940455

MED024000MEDICAL / Education & Training

!Wagner Wolf Publishing!

P.O. Box 63 South Orange, NJ 07079-9998

Visit our website at www.wagnerwolf.com

Follow us on http://twitter.com/#!/PreMedAdvice

Read our blog: www.WagnerWolf.wordpress.com

Watch our videos: http://www.youtube.com/user/TheWagnerTV

ACKNOWLEDGMENTS

Through Christ all things are possible

Wagner Wolf Publishing, LLC would like to thank everyone who played a part in this book's success. *So You Wanna Be A Doctor?? The Untold Stories of Medical, Dental, and Veterinary Residents* owes a great deal to the chapter contributors:

Shermian P. Daniel, M.D.
Adonia H. Dibbell, M.D.
Elo C. Adibe, D.M.D.
Miguel A. Coba, M.D.
Richard H. Huggins, M.D.
Yvelisse N. Suarez, M.D.
L. Efua Essandoh, M.D.
Joya S. Griffin, D.V.M.
Trevor H. Atherley, M.D.
Leon S. Dick, M.D.

A special thanks to Pamela Charles, Antoinette Odom, Nathalie Green, Phillip Charles, Marva Scotland, Cecilia Babb, and Paakwesi Ashon

Last but not least, thanks to YOU for picking up this book! We have worked very hard to compile great stories and essential resources for you – learn all you can and put the information to good use!

TABLE OF CONTENTS

ACKNOWLEDGMENTS vi

INTRODUCTION ix

ABBREVIATIONS & DEFINITIONS xi

ANESTHESIA .... *"Hmmm – That's Weird ...Making It Through Anesthesia and All Of Life's Interruptions"*.................Shermian P. Daniel, M.D. 3

PHYSICAL MEDICINE & REHABILITATION ....
..............."*Finding Yourself In Medicine*" ....
.... Miguel A. Coba, M.D.....................55

PATHOLOGY .... *"You're Not A Real Doctor*........... Yvelisse N. Suarez, M.D............69

VETERINARY MEDICINE .... *"Veterinarians: Doctors Who Treat* More *Than Just One Species"* .... Joya S. Griffin, D.V.M. 117

DENTISTRY ...."*You Don't Have To Brush Your Teeth - Just The Ones You Want To Keep"* ....Elo C. Adibe, D.M.D. 130

PEDIATRICS .... *"Life Is Good...Now"*................ Adonia H. Dibbell, M.D. 143

DERMATOLOGY .... *"Is It A Rash?"*......... Richard H. Huggins, M.D. 153

OBSTETRICS & GYNECOLOGY .... *"You May Encounter Many Defeats, But You Must Not Be Defeated"* ... . L. Efua Essandoh, M.D. ....…....167

CARDIOLOGY/SURGERY.... *"Been There, Done That"* Trevor H. Atherley, M.D., P.A. and Leon S. Dick, M.D., P.A 189

CODE BLUE .... *"20 Do's and Don'ts For Surviving An Emergency Situation"*........... Shermian P. Daniel, M.D. and Richard S. Daniel ....….....199

GENERAL INFORMATION .... *"Essential Residency Resources"* ....…... Shermian P. Daniel, M.D. and Richard S. Daniel …...203

INTRODUCTION
By Richard S. Daniel

I always wanted to know what it took to become a highly respected doctor or physician in today's society of rigid standards and high expectations. I knew you had to be smart so I didn't want to sound dumb by asking a simple question such as, 'what do you have to do to become a doctor?'.

Ever since watching the Huxtables on the Cosby Show or hearing a parent ask a child what they wanted to be when they grew up, a doctor or lawyer always seemed to be the preferred occupations to strive for. Almost 100% of the time being a doctor was suggested first. Being a physician or any specialist in the medical field is one of the most sought after and prestigious positions, and consequently one of the hardest goals to achieve.

As children grow, they become teenagers and consider their future careers after high school more seriously. The other cliché career paths such as policeman, firefighter, or teacher then become more realistic options. School guidance counselors are not fully informed regarding the steps involved to become a part of the medical profession. Parents are even less aware of the process and are usually not in a very informed position to give advice on this matter to their child.

In my search on the topic I was never able to find one reference point that could answer my most basic questions in a simplified manner. I also wanted to know how the experience was first hand from someone who recently went through it - not from someone who only read about it in a book, or from someone who went through their journey twenty or thirty years ago when standards and technologies were vastly different from what they are today.

I am grateful that the authors and contributors of this book were willing and able to share their experiences and insight with us. This allows someone from the outside looking in to get a better in-depth understanding of how to get into the medical profession and what to expect during their journey. I hope you gather lots of useful information from this book and come back for more exciting titles in the future!

...Before We Get Started
Abbreviations & Definitions...

Medicine can be very complex - especially when you don't understand the language! What follows is a list of some common abbreviations and terms that may help you while reading this book:

■■

Internship: A one year paid position for a physician who has finished medical school, but not the more specialized training of a residency program. An intern may or may not have a medical license or a D.E.A. number to dispense controlled substances.

Residency: The stage of graduate medical education which takes place after graduation from medical school and the completion of an internship. Resident physicians practice medicine in a variety of specialties under the supervision of a fully trained and licensed physician, usually in a clinic or hospital.

Fellowship: The medical training that may be done after residency for even more expertise in a given field. Usually lasting more than one year, a fellowship can be done in many fields like cardiology, sports medicine, or pain medicine.

PGY - Post-Graduate Year: This tells how many years it has been since a physician graduated from medical school. A person who is at a PGY-4 level, for example, graduated 4 years ago and could be at a more advanced stage of his/her residency with more responsibilities and a slightly higher salary.

CA - Clinical Anesthesia: A term used when referring to anesthesia residents. It is usually followed by a number – 1, 2, or 3 – depending on the resident's position during an anesthesia training program.

Attending: A person who has completed residency training and is now in charge of a health care team. He/She is 'the boss' and will lead rounds with residents, hold teaching sessions throughout the day, and be ultimately responsible for all of the patients on a given team.

Rounds: Each day, health care teams walk around the hospital and discuss the patients admitted to their medical service. All information about a patient is discussed in detail, from vital signs, physical findings, overnight events, and current therapies. Rounds are led by an attending physician, and can include residents, medical students, nurses, therapists, and even administrators.

Consult: A consult is a discussion (or consultation) with another health care provider regarding a patient. For instance, a patient may be admitted to the Family Medicine service for complications related to diabetes, but a consult may be placed to an ophthalmologist regarding the patient's blurred vision.

AAMC/AACOM - American Association of Medical Colleges/American Association of Colleges of Osteopathic Medicine: These are the only two national medical college associations in the United States. They support education, research, and patient care activities in our country.

ACGME - American College of Graduate Medical Education: This is a private, non-profit council that evaluates and accredits medical residency programs in the United States.

USMLE - United States Medical Licensing Exam: This is a three-part licensing examination that is required to receive a license to practice medicine in the U.S.A. It is taken during medical school and residency.

MCAT - Medical College Admissions Test: This is a day-long test required by all American medical schools for admission. It focuses on biological/physical sciences, organic/inorganic chemistry, and writing/reading skills.

OB-GYN - Obstetrics and Gynecology: A physician who has successfully completed specialized education and training in the management of women's health, pregnancy, labor, and the time period following childbirth.

HCP - Health Care Provider: A person who delivers proper, systematic, and professional medical care to any individual in need.

ACLS - Advanced Cardiac Life Support: This refers to a set of clinical interventions for the treatment of cardiac arrest and other life threatening medical emergencies. It must be administered by a highly trained person.

BLS - Basic Life Support: This is a level of medical care used for patients with life-threatening illness or injury until they get full care in a hospital setting. It is administered by trained personnel, often times without medical equipment.

DNR - Do Not Resuscitate: This is an order placed on a patient's medical chart that tells medical personnel not to perform cardiopulmonary resuscitation if the patient's breathing or heartbeat stop.

H&P - History and Physical: This is a list of information gathered by a health care professional about a patient's medical problems, family health, vital signs, organ-specific health, and more. It is usually done during a visit with a doctor.

ICU - Intensive Care Unit: Also known as a critical care unit, this is a specialized hospital department that delivers care to the sickest, most complicated and challenging patients. There are many types, including neonatal, surgical, and neurological.

OR - Operating Room: This is where surgical operations and procedures are carried out.   Staffed by doctors, nurses, and technicians, operating rooms must be sterile, and well equipped to handle any medical situation.

P.A. - Professional Association: If you see this after M.D. in a person's title, it is simply a legal term to describe a separate legal entity and protect individuals from lawsuits. This is not to be confused with physician assistant, which has the same abbreviation.

"Hmmm – That's Weird... Making It Through Anesthesia and All Of Life's Interruptions"

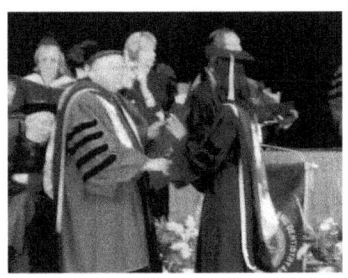

Shermian P. Daniel, M.D.
PGY-3, CA-1, Department of Anesthesiology
Mayo Clinic/Mayo School of Graduate Medical
Education, Jacksonville, FL

IN THIS CHAPTER...

*What does it take to make it through college?

* How can I get into medical school?

* What types of activities look best on one's resume?

* What does one do during an internship program?

* What is the life of an anesthesia resident like?

* How does one deal with unexpected setbacks in medicine?

I had a golden weekend, and I wanted to make the most of it. That means that I was on call at the hospital Thursday night, and so by noon on Friday, I was already home, packing my things, and heading back out the door. I grabbed my favorite party clothes, had a bite to eat, and gave myself a final once-over in the mirror. After a quick trip to the car rental spot, my weekend of fun had officially begun! The music-filled ride from Jacksonville, FL to Atlanta, GA didn't take long, and after getting lost once, I arrived at my friend's house.

Once I put my bags down, the first thing on my agenda was food!! I was starving, but luckily, a local fast food joint came to my rescue. I ordered a burger and a drink, went back to my friend's house, and lounged lazily on the couch. An hour of television surfing went by; I then realized that I was tired (being on call takes a toll on you, after all). I sat up, turned around, and put my feet on the ground. No big deal - we do this a thousand times a day, but this time was different for me. My right leg felt like it was 'falling asleep'. Again, no big deal, except that it persisted, regardless of how much I shook it out. "Hmmm - that's weird" is all I said to myself before retreating upstairs for a long, peaceful slumber.

Morning. I sat up in bed and put my feet on the ground. Right leg was still slightly numb, but I was too eager to party and let loose to really care. At breakfast, I noticed that my tongue felt a little weird. It felt like I had burned it; I couldn't really taste anything. I brushed this off as a probable burn from scarfing down last night's fast food and continued on. I didn't notice any other symptoms, and the rest of the weekend was blissful fun - a much needed rejuvenation before starting a grueling month in the intensive care unit (ICU).

Over the next three weeks - you guessed it - the numbness in my right leg did not disappear. In fact, it got worse, even spreading to my left leg. I was certain that this was going to be a self-limited process that would go away on its own with no lasting effects. So when my tongue, bottom lip, and the entire left side of my face went numb, I kept working. When I couldn't remember the lyrics to my favorite songs or sing along in the car without getting tongue-tied, I figured I just had too much on my mind. When my vision got blurry and I had trouble merging into traffic when driving, I thought it was simple fatigue from long hospital hours. You would think that limping through halls and having to hold onto walls for balance would set off an alarm in my head, but I didn't take action until my mother and brother heard of my symptoms and urged me to visit my doctor.

I woke up extra early one Tuesday morning and rounded on all of my ICU patients. I looked up overnight vital signs and lab results, did patient exams, and wrote all of my notes for the day. I made sure that everyone was relatively stable and that there was nothing pressing that I had to do. I then sheepishly approached the ICU fellow and let him know that I had to leave for a doctor's appointment. I felt bad for leaving, but promised to return when my visit was over, even though all of my work for the day had been taken care of. He let me go with no argument - he had watched me stumble around the hospital over the last few days, just like all the other residents, attendings, and nurses.

I drove slowly to the clinic, careful not to let my blurred vision lead to an interstate pile-up. I sat in the waiting room a few minutes before my doctor called me in for an examination. As soon as she saw my attempt to walk and heard the accompanying story, she had a hunch as to what could be wrong. She got on the phone with the Neurology and Radiology departments, then rushed me off to the MRI scanner. They made me undress and started an IV in order to administer contrast, a visualizing substance for the test. They gave me earplugs to block out all the noise that was to come, then laid me on a hard stretcher. An hour later, the machine stopped churning, and I was released to await the results.

Upon returning to the ICU at my hospital, I was informed that rounds with our attending were over for the day, and I was free to go home. Since it was still early, I happily drove home and broke out all of my books for an exciting day of studying thrombotic thrombocytopenic purpura. I had just settled onto my couch when the phone rang…

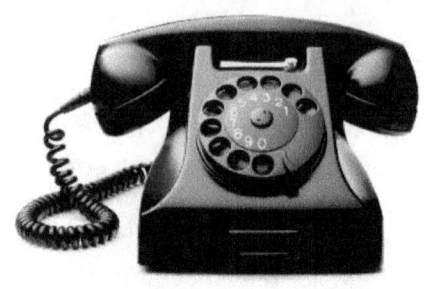

"Hello?"

"Hi, Shermian? This is your doctor. I'm calling about your test results."

"Oh, wow - that was quick. Is everything alright?"

"Well, not too long after you left, I got a phone call from the doctor who read your MRI. We discussed it, then got on the phone with our colleagues from the Neurology department."

"Okay. What did they say?"

"Well...they saw some worrisome changes on the scan of your brain, and would like you to come in for some more testing. It doesn't look like a tumor, but I am recommending that you be urgently admitted to the hospital right now so we can get to the bottom of this. I think you should pack up some clothes in an overnight bag, and make arrangements to come over to the hospital. Are you alright?"

Whew.

"Yeah, I'm okay, I guess - this is just so...sudden. Worrisome changes, huh? You said it's not a tumor, right? Urgently admitted? Uhhh, so who do I ask for when I get there? How long will I be in the hospital?"

That conversation continued and I got all the details I needed. I packed a bag like she suggested - I even brought some books, since I was behind in my reading. Next, I sat on the edge of my bed and called my mother. We called my father on three-way and I broke the news to them. I had been handling the news just fine when my doctor told me, but couldn't even get the sentence out when talking to my parents. I finally broke down crying and could not utter one word on the phone. I know it must have freaked them out since they had no idea of what had happened that day. I tried to hold it together, but couldn't help the tears - it suddenly dawned on me that this could be something serious - something I certainly had never experienced in all of my healthy life. What is going on? What could the problem be? Am I going to die? Is there something I did to bring this on? Why did I wait so long to seek help? What about work? What is my life going to be like from this point on?

Before we continue down that grim path, let me first tell you how I got to this point...

∎∎

1989. 4th grade. That was the first time I can recall feeling smart - like I had potential in life. My teacher that year made all the difference. From giving me extra class projects to work on, making learning a little more fun for the whole class, and his total confidence in my academic abilities, the spark of interest in education was set off in me. I tried harder, paid more attention, and sought opportunities to challenge myself. Now most children don't take the time to plan their futures in full detail at the ripe old age of 9, but I guess I was strange in that way. Even as a small child, I contemplated how things worked on a fundamental level, so I thought that science or engineering could be for me. I admired the strong intellectuals in my world, so I read voraciously in order to be like the teachers, lawyers, artists, and activists around me. I was a real busy-body - constantly doing after-school programs, yearning for travel, and joining school clubs. I did everything from sports to performing arts, church and civic activities, so I knew that I wasn't afraid of hard work or service to my community. I looked into engineering and research, but they failed to capture my imagination. Years later, I noticed that I had a strange interest in horror movies, blood & guts, and all things gruesome, so I thought of a way to incorporate that onto my list of possible career choices. Add all those things up and survey says...medicine was definitely my first and only real choice.

I liked school. I graduated from Columbia High School in Maplewood, NJ with an array of wonderful experiences under my belt – everything from a Latin language club, track-n-field, church youth group, cheerleading, and the Prom Committee. I eased into college life with no problem after this. My parents chose The Johns Hopkins University in Baltimore, MD for my college education. And yes, you read that correctly – they *made* me go there against my will! I had so many other schools (ahem, party schools) that I wanted to explore, but since I wanted a top-notch school with a long record of getting students into medical school, my folks insisted on JHU. I argued, cried, and pouted up until move-in day, then prepared to say goodbye to any chance of fun or normalcy in the future. I couldn't believe they were making this decision *for* me – wasn't I supposed to be an adult with the power to make my own choices in life? I felt cheated, and I let everyone know of my discontent.

As is often the case though, parents know best, and I ended up having a fabulous time at a fabulous institution. I complained until the last minute, but even I couldn't stop the excitement from creeping in when it was time to head down to Baltimore. The move-in process was painless that first day, and the Black Student Union (BSU) hosted a welcome reception for all eager, young freshmen. Our parents were kept busy at their own functions, leading to the tearful good-byes when move-in day was over. There weren't many tears from me – I was off to my first Student Council party that night! I met kids from New York and New Jersey who were just like me, and even laid eyes on one or two good looking guys! I partied with students from Ohio, California, Texas, and Washington; I walked across every inch of the campus, and stayed up for hours just talking and laughing. I was loving life, and enjoying my new-found freedom.

My classmates and I sailed through Orientation week, choosing classes and becoming acquainted with the student organizations looking for new members. I chose a Biology major and Spanish minor early in the semester. I could have chosen to major in Public Health, Neuroscience, or Engineering like many of my friends did, but I genuinely liked Biology, so I chose that and prepared for the work ahead. I worked my way through Introduction to Chemistry, got creative in Introduction to Fiction and Poetry, and toiled away in Calculus II. I didn't like Physics or Organic Chemistry as much (not many students do!), but with a few sleepless nights, I got through them also.

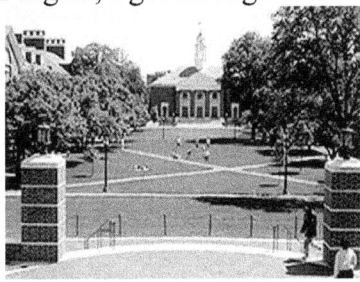

The Black Student Union (BSU) offered my first taste of real leadership in college, for I was named co-chairwoman of the Black History Month committee during my second year. My friend and I worked endlessly to secure speakers, organize banquets, put on step-shows, and provide lots of good food. We went above and beyond the norm in order to make that month truly unforgettable. Our activities were all fun, informative, creative, and inspiring. What resulted was a flawless February, full of spectacular events – we were the talk of the campus after the festivities ended! It felt good to have our hard work pay off – we were on our way to bright and successful careers, and this was just the beginning!

After that, I couldn't get enough of organizational involvement, and became active in so many varied things. I was vice-president, then president of the BSU. I pledged Delta Sigma Theta Sorority, Inc., the second oldest fraternal organization comprised of African-American women who are passionate about scholarship and service. I mentored in and became co-chairperson for the Mentoring Assistance Peer Program, a wonderful group dedicated to helping multicultural freshmen adjust to life on a college campus and excel in their studies. I joined the Hopkins chapter of the Minority Association of Pre-Health Students (MAPS), and traveled to Nashville, TN for a six-week intensive summer program (MMEP, the Minority Medical

Education Program) meant to expose students to life in the health professions and give them a head-start when it came to medical school applications. I also worked with the Multi-Ethnic Students at Hopkins (MESH), National Association for the Advancement of Colored People (NAACP), JHUnity club, and Caribbean Cultural Society (CCS) – anything that would look good on my resume. I told you that I was always a busy-body, and it only got worse in college.

I loved to party, hang with friends, and attend meetings. There weren't many functions that I stayed away from, whether it was a dance extravaganza for CultureFest, or a round table discussion with the Inter-Asian Council. If there was free food available or an interesting movie being shown, I was there. If some folks were going on a road trip, more than likely, I was the first one there with bags packed. My studies, surprisingly, were not flourishing as much as my social calendar during this period, so I finally took a long, hard look at my priorities. I decided to once again become the student I had been in high school, when good grades came effortlessly. No medical school would want me with B's and C's on my transcript, so by my junior year of college, I buckled down and took up residence at the Milton S. Eisenhower library on campus. I attended every class lecture, took meticulous notes, then schlepped to the library's quiet lower level to organize my notes and absorb the material. I started feeling good about my classes, and believe it or not, I got excited about learning Developmental Biology, Reproductive Physiology, and Virology. Next I began close work with our pre-professional advisors to create a list of potential schools I would apply to. I took a mini-MCAT preparation course and practiced questions & essay responses as often as I could. The MCAT (Medical College Admission Test) scores I received were not as high as I wanted them to be, but they were good enough to not require that I retake them. That was a relief for me, because the MCAT has been known to be the downfall for many, many students.

The summer after my junior year was a good one; that was when I secured an internship in Manhattan for a Methodist missionary foundation. While here, I worked on my med school application, and I narrowed my application choices to schools in the northeast. After the choices were made, I then started on the AMCAS (American Medical College Application Service) process. Each day I did painstakingly detailed work on the online forms and documents. I wrote and rewrote my personal statement, while getting lots of help from my professors and mentors. I listed each of my extra-curricular activities so they sounded as impressive as possible. I double-checked everything on the application twice, then held my breath while I pushed the send button.

One September day, I was surprised by a letter offering my first medical school interview. It came sooner than expected, but I wasted no time in scheduling that precious meeting. I cleared my schedule and bought my Greyhound ticket in order to travel to Newark, NJ early in October. My last meeting with our pre-professional advisors left me with lots of hope; I felt good and very, very excited. Upon my arrival at New Jersey Medical School (NJMS), I was greeted by a medical student and brought up to the admissions office for my interview. My nerves were evident that day, but my interviewer put me at ease right away and started a pleasant conversation about my accomplishments and goals. We talked about what I had done in college, what I wanted to do in medical school, and why I was so passionate about the field. I didn't escape without having to explain my less than spectacular grades during freshman and sophomore year, but instead of badgering me about them, we discussed how I had turned things around and become a more focused and mature applicant. An hour flew by, then he released me to take a tour of the grounds. I loved everything I heard about the school, and felt a great sense of warmth from the students who stopped to chat with me. People seemed relaxed and happy to be studying there. Everyone I saw was hard at work, but none too busy to answer my questions. There were even fliers and bulletins announcing lots of fun-sounding activities (a wonderful plus for me!). By the end of that day, my excitement about medicine was reinforced and I looked forward to my other interviews. I did go on several more interviews, but never felt at home like I did at NJMS. That was important to me, since I would be spending inordinate amounts of time at any medical school that I chose. When acceptance letters came around later that spring I was able to place the letter from NJMS on top of the pile. I breathed a huge sigh of relief, and did a quick dance of joy. After this, I returned to having some fun before I graduated from college and left my glorious days at Johns Hopkins behind. Disclaimer: JHU is NOT a party school by any stretch of the imagination, but *I* had my fun – go figure…

Medical school started off on a wonderful note. Proud that I had accomplished one major goal (getting into med school), I was eager to accomplish lots more. NJMS sponsored a summer program for students to begin med school work early. Needless to say, I took advantage of the F.I.R.S.T. (Freshman Introduction to Resources and Skills Training) program. Here, we got to take courses in anatomy and meet the students who would be our lifeline over the next four years. We got to work on cadavers and learned about the organs, blood vessels, and nerves that help the body function. We memorized bones, joints, and ligaments until we couldn't learn anymore, and made up silly songs to help recall the information. I partied that summer (of course!), got to know the Newark area, and prepared for what was to come as a med student.

My improved study habits came with me to medical school, and I found a classmate to review notes with every day. We made sure that we caught every word the professor said, then made sure that it all made some sense. I felt good for the first few weeks; unfortunately, I got a rude awakening the day before my first biochemistry quiz. My study partner and I glimpsed at some sample questions and realized that we didn't know how to answer them. Apparently just *looking* at notes was not enough, and we were not prepared to be quizzed on any of the material. We agreed that an all-nighter was called for, and after a long night of cramming, we emerged confident that we had finally mastered the covered material. We both passed that quiz, but from that moment on, my study habits were dramatically improved, again. I spent hours everyday reviewing notes, writing outlines, reading textbook passages, and quizzing myself on the subjects. I could not move to a new page until I knew the facts forwards and backwards, and this continued through Genetics, Histology, and Microbiology. Other students praised our study techniques, and we inspired several others to join us in cementing the material every night. We each had our preferred rooms to study in, and even had seats that we felt lucky in. If you were looking for me during first or second year of med school, you knew where to find me, for I was at the school all the time - days, nights, weekends, and holidays.

At this time, I applied for a dual-degree program that would allow me to get a Masters degree in Public Health along with a medical degree. I always knew that I liked medicine, but also wanted a way to do my share of community service. I wanted to eradicate health care disparities, study the diseases that disproportionately affected people of color, and work on cures for the ills that claim the lives of too many. I was accepted into the M.P.H.

program at NJMS and started to take classes. I found them to be easy. We crunched numbers and learned biostatistical formulas that could be applied to scientific research. I passed my first class without a problem but got discouraged when it seemed that all my classes would center on statistics, and not the large scale epidemiology that I wanted. I wanted to one day work at the Centers for Disease Control (CDC) or don one of those big biohazard suits seen in movies like *Outbreak* or *The Andromeda Strain*. Formulating null hypotheses and performing ANOVA tests wasn't my idea of fun. Not wanting to wade through those beginner classes, I abandoned my public health studies after one year. I probably should not have since it was a good opportunity, but oh well – my impatience won in this case.

Physiology, Nutrition, and Neuroscience came and went, then it was time for a summer break. I didn't want to be idle with my time, so I found two programs to participate in. The first was sponsored by the Mayo Clinic, a world renowned institution - a leader in medical advancements and first-class health care. They flew a handful of students to their main campus in Rochester, MN to spend three weeks shadowing doctors in different specialties. We got to work with surgeons, primary care doctors, and obstetricians. We had seminars on improving communication with patients and leading health care teams. I had a great time at this program, and kept in touch with its participants and administrators throughout medical school. The next thing I did that summer was a Neuroscience program for local high school students sponsored by NJMS. I was selected to be a tutor for those students and we split them into teams that heard lectures from practicing neurosurgeons, developed their own research projects, and took trips to science museums in the area. That was a very fulfilling experience, and it reenergized me to continue on the path to graduation.

In my second year of medical school, I continued hard work in the classroom in classes like Pathology and Pharmacology, but also added some more leadership to my curriculum vitae. I was elected president of the NJMS chapter of the Student National Medical Association (SNMA), and hit the ground running. This is the nation's oldest group dedicated to the needs of medical students and communities of color, and I was honored to be a part of it. Not only did we elect a chapter vice-president, treasurer, and secretary, but also formed an auxiliary board, filled with students who would lead our community service, political advocacy, social event, and college student initiatives. I devoted so much time and energy to that organization, and couldn't be happier with what we accomplished. We mentored students, fundraised in creative ways, formed amazing study groups, and supported lots of Newark health fairs. We put together a large Pre-Health Leadership Symposium for undergraduate students, and co-hosted a gathering of the nation's only Black transplant surgeons. Our chapter banquet that year was a classy and cultured way to honor those making a difference in the Newark area, and gave us a chance to relax after working so hard all year round. We were a close knit group throughout the year, and were rewarded with the region's Chapter of the Year honor during the annual SNMA national conference in New Orleans. Words cannot express my gratitude for that organization and the highlights it brought to my life! I worked on the national SNMA membership committee the next year, and worked with the American Medical Women's Association. I was on the Student Assistance Campus Committee, and helped the babies in Project Pediatrics – all great for my resume and residency application!

Studying for USMLE Step 1 took up the rest of my second year. The United States Medical Licensing Examination (USMLE) consists of three parts – the first 8-

hour test is taken after second year, the second two-part test is done during fourth year, and the third 8-hour test is done during residency. These tests cover all types of medical information and require intense studying (and heaps of registration money!). They have multiple choice questions, computer based medical scenarios, and actual patient interaction evaluations. A passing score on the USMLE tests is required for graduation from most medical schools, promotion during some residency programs, and the granting of a medical license to dispense medication and safely care for patients. NJMS offered a Kaplan course to help us prepare for Step 1. There was also a school-sponsored review course to help us with Step 2. For Step 3, I had graduated from NJMS, so I was on my own for its preparation. Along with the review courses, I also needed study groups, flashcards, sample questions, and lots of prayer to pass these tests! I did pass each test on the first try – my scores weren't off the charts, but just like with the MCAT years earlier, it was good enough to move forward with. I did a one-week program at the Mayo Clinic's Scottsdale, AZ site after I took Step 1. Another way to get a head start when it came to surviving rotations, choosing specialties, and getting accepted into residencies; I enjoyed it and took lots of lessons away from that short time.

Third year was surprisingly a lot of fun. Gone were the days of studying a book for 12 hours each day – third year meant hands-on patient care. We were done learning about the fundamentals of medical science; now we focused on how body systems could be devastated by disease. We traveled to different area hospitals and met lots of different attendings. We learned how to administer fluids, perform gynecologic and urologic exams, and do full exams on newborns. We assisted in various surgeries, assessed for mental health disease, and took care of critical patients. Rounds with residents and attendings, where we discussed all the patients admitted to our service, were great ways to see connections among lifestyle, genetics, health care access, and proper medical care. I'll admit it though – the internal medicine rotation was pretty scary to me that year. You have to know about an endless number of diseases and treatments. You have to deal with lots of patients – old ones, sick ones, mentally unstable ones, and downright mean ones. Medicine attendings can be very demanding, and the first time I had to present a patient's history entirely from memory, I almost convinced myself to call out sick that day! As with other rotations, I got through it. The residents were excellent and I was so proud that I impressed them with my work ethic and fund of knowledge. When third year came to a close, my classmates and I felt so accomplished! We were absorbing high volumes of information, impressing our patient care teams every day, and coming closer to that glorious day when a medical degree would be ours.

Fourth year was even more fun, because we got to choose our own schedules for the most part. Everyone had to rotate through Internal Medicine, Family Medicine, Obstetrics and Gynecology, Pediatrics, Surgery, and Psychiatry in third year; in fourth year, we had to do Neurology, Physical Medicine and Rehabilitation, Urology, and Emergency Medicine. After that, we could revisit the areas that interested us most, or explore the specialties that intrigued us as possible specialty choices. I did rotations in Anesthesia, Pathology, Radiology, Medical Genetics, and International Medicine. Some of these were visiting clerkships, where I traveled to hospitals in Jacksonville, FL, Atlanta, GA, and Washington, D.C. to see how their programs worked. I also studied abroad with two classmates for a month in Oaxaca, Mexico through the Child Family Health International (CFHI) organization. Here, we got true hands-on experience – both culturally and medically. We observed how health care was run in large hospitals and private medical offices. I saw acupuncture and other alternative medicine treatments performed. We took excursions to remote areas, sat in on advanced Spanish language courses, and ate some delicious authentic food. It was truly an extraordinary way to end my time as a medical student.

But before I can move on, I have to figure out what the next step will be, right? Starting early in fourth year, I began the application process for residency. Not everyone has to do a residency program after medical school, but if you want specialized training in medical fields like pediatrics or pathology, you must apply for, be accepted to, and graduate from an accredited residency program. This can take three years all the way up to eight years, but this is the time when great doctors are born and learn the skills that will stay with them throughout their career.

During second year, in Pharmacology class, I first became interested in Anesthesiology. I thought the gases and local anesthetics used in that field sounded like fun substances to work with, so I tried to learn more. Imagine a simple, colorless vapor that can put a person into a safe, but deep sleep during surgery. How cool would it be to work with powerful liquids that can quickly and effectively numb up any body part, big or small. When I found out that there were lots of hands-on procedures that anesthesiologists perform everyday, I wanted to be a part of it. Life saving intubations, tracheostomies, spinals, epidurals, and triple lumen catheter placements would be mine to do all the time! And when I looked at the excitement, adventure, lifestyle, and salary associated with it, I knew that I definitely wanted to pursue a residency program in Anesthesia.

Therefore, my first visiting clerkship in fourth year was to the Mayo Clinic program in Jacksonville, FL. It was a great month, of course – lots of teaching, interesting cases, and fun residents to hang out with. The city seemed cool – right next to the beach, good weather, and laid back living (unlike the busy northeast). In addition to this program, I applied to and interviewed at about 6 programs along the east coast that fall. Interviews were fun, although very tiring. There was nothing special about my interviews – lots of travel, and lots of the same questions over and over. I didn't get any of the crazy interviews that are out there – no one asked me outrageous personal questions or did anything extremely offensive.

Ranking programs was more stressful than anticipated, however. Of all the programs that offered an interview, you could then rank the ones you were interested in. The programs would rank the students they wanted to join them, and so, 'rank lists' were made. If the program you listed as number one also ranked you as their number one pick, then you were going to that program for residency. It gets tricky if you aren't dealing with the number one student or program, but for the most part, it all works out. Rank lists are submitted in February; computer match algorithms then take all the information and pair students with programs. In mid-March, all graduating students pursuing residency receive a letter in the mail simply stating, "Congratulations, you have matched", or the opposite if the rank process didn't work out in their favor. For those who did not match into a program, they can then 'scramble', where they contact programs that did not fill all of their residency positions, and negotiate for admittance. Three days later, everyone gathers for Match Day – the students who matched originally, and the ones who successfully negotiated into a program. Everyone is handed an envelope, inside of which is the name and location of the program you matched into. NJMS had a large, fun-filled celebration with professors, administrators, families, and newscasters invited. I tore my envelope open with no hesitation and was pleased to see the name of my number one choice listed: The Mayo School of Graduate Medical Education for a four-year residency in anesthesia.

After that day, there was a lot of partying going on – we were all elated to have victoriously navigated through four years of medical school. There were some nail-biting times, some tears, and mishaps, but that was all behind us. We finished our rotations for school, went to organizational conferences, attended award ceremonies, and had lots of graduation parties. These students really were my lifeline, and I was extremely proud to share this accomplishment with them. And even more exciting than graduation was the time in residency ahead, where we would learn unprecedented amounts about taking care of patients and critical situations, and master the specialties of our choosing. I, for one, couldn't wait!!

Alright. You may be thinking that I'm living a fairy tale, and things aren't as easy as I make it seem. I know this, but this is *my* experience. I knew what I wanted from an early age, and did what was necessary to make it happen. I sought advice when necessary, and always had a plan ready to go. I was two steps ahead of the game at all times, and made sure to enjoy the ride while it lasted. Other stories may be fraught with difficulties and hardships, but not mine. Not yet, at least…

Armed with my match letter and the ton of paperwork that was mailed to me in the following weeks, I headed off to Florida to start my new life. First things first - I needed a place to stay. My parents and I flew down and got a realtor to show us suitable properties. I knew that I wanted to buy a house, since I would be in Jacksonville for at least 4 years. We saw several places, then I settled on a gorgeous townhouse 10 minutes from my hospital. It was three-stories, in a quiet development, with great amenities, and a posh outdoor mall next door. It was a little pricey, but now that I was making real money, I was willing to take on the mortgage. It's not big-shot 'doctor money', mind you, but my resident salary was definitely enough.

Orientation week was good. PowerPoint presentations on hospital policies, tours of hospital and clinic grounds, and ID photo sessions took place. We took basic life support (BLS) and advanced cardiac life support (ACLS) classes. Computers and passwords were assigned, and finally, we were handed our white coats and pagers. After years of wearing a short white coat to denote that I was a medical student, now I had my very own long coat – two, actually! My program's name was stitched on the lapel, and the pockets were just waiting for me to fill them up with books and papers. It was finally official – we really were doctors, with the white coats and pagers reminding us that we had paid our dues and gained admittance to a very special club of professionals. At night during orientation, the residents took us out for happy hours, dinners, barbecues, and other get-togethers. We all shared our fears about starting residency and the added responsibilities it would bring. No longer could we say "I don't know the answer to that question, I'm just a medical student" – patient lives now depended on our vigilance and professionalism. It was a huge weight on our shoulders, but nothing we couldn't handle without common sense, proper guidance, and lots more studying.

My first rotation was in the anesthesia department. This was a piece of cake, because I had already rotated there as a medical student. I didn't have to take overnight call, or do many of the procedures that residents are expected to do - except endotracheal intubations and venipunctures, of course!

I'll skip ahead to the next month, my first Internal Medicine rotation as a resident. This is the rotation where you take care of the sick patients admitted to the hospital. They aren't the ones who have just had babies or surgeries, and they aren't in critical condition like those in the intensive care unit. These patients may have uncontrolled blood sugar or blood pressure, various types of infections, pain issues, strokes, or heart disorders. There are limitless processes that can land someone in the hospital, and as the intern (first year resident), it is your job to interview and examine the patient daily, keep up with their vital signs and blood work, know what treatments they're on or tests they're scheduled for, and document all of this in daily progress notes. Also important is to learn about their disease for discussions during rounds, and to formulate plans for their return to health and discharge from the hospital. It can be a busy day, a long day, and a frustrating day, or it can be a peaceful day where all of your patients are cooperative, you get your work done with no hassles or setbacks, and you learn a valuable new piece of medical information. At first, most of my days were long and busy. I hadn't yet mastered the computer system, so it took forever to access patient information and write my admission history & physicals (h&p's). I didn't know my way around the hospital, so if someone sent me to the pathology lab or neuroradiology suite, I wouldn't know where to go. I was still a bit unsure of myself as a new doctor, so when I had to call another medical team or a specialist for help or advice about a patient, I didn't quite know what to say. The first time I was paged by a nurse with a question about a patient, I listened intently, then told her I would call her back. I then ran down the hall, looked up dosing recommendations for the anti-psychotic drug Haldol, and got back to the phone three minutes later. I told that nurse that it was okay to give her sundowning patient his prescribed dose of the drug, for he often became uninhibited at night time. I felt silly after this encounter, because all she wanted to know was whether she could give a drug that had already been written for and given the evening prior. Oooops!

Luckily, this flustered feeling always goes away quickly. The feeling of not knowing enough and the fear of making a fatal mistake doesn't last too long. After one or two weeks, you find yourself getting good at the routine. You can actually answer questions when someone pages you for information. You can admit a patient and dictate your notes in less and less time. You can survive overnight call and all the craziness that happens when the sun goes down and the regular hospital staff goes home. You are cramped into small call rooms, and are awakened every hour to deal with patients that are itching, in pain, or giving nurses a hard time. You learn to deal with death and near death experiences. When that code blue announcement is suddenly made over the loudspeaker, you bolt through the hallways to the location of the commotion. You assess the situation and find out where you can be of service. You remove your white coat, roll up your sleeves, and take over for the exhausted resident performing CPR (cardio-pulmonary-resuscitation) on an 83-year old man with pulmonary edema (fluid in the lungs) and a poorly functioning heart. You look through the patient's chart to find out what medications he is on and to ensure that he does not have a DNR (Do Not Resuscitate) order on file. You familiarize yourself with his history so you can brief the ICU team when they arrive to transport him downstairs for further care. You do the necessary paperwork and collect yourself before returning to *your* assigned patients and the examinations you were in the middle of doing with them. You go home later and read about the arrhythmias (abnormal heart beats) that can lead to pulmonary edema, so that the next time something like that happens, you'll be prepared and informed.

During my first year of residency, I got good at the medical stuff. I was diligent, hard-working, respectful, intelligent, easy to work with, and skilled with my hands. I got along with people and didn't take shortcuts in order to finish the work day early or avoid unpleasant tasks. My attendings seemed to like me, and the other interns seemed to like working with me. I felt good each day when I stepped out of the hospital and sauntered towards my car. I would roll the windows down and let that warm Florida breeze keep me company during the short drive home. I'd get home, pick up my mail, feed my cat, grab some microwavable burritos or a peanut butter sandwich, then settle in front of the t.v. Admittedly, I did not study as much as I could have, but I did a little each day and I picked up the pace when it was time to study for Step 3 or prepare a presentation for work. My eating habits left much to be desired, but I rationalized it by saying that I wasn't eating fast food and I would hit the gym near my house a few times each week. On weekends I would head out to the thrift shops and antique stores that always had unique items for purchase. I would meet up with colleagues to walk along the beach or take in a movie. I went to a nearby church to sing songs and hear good sermons. Many times, I would book a last minute flight and jaunt off to see old friends in Baltimore, Chicago, Los Angeles, or anywhere else I fancied.

Loneliness unfortunately played a big part in my Florida experience. I have always loved spending time with friends and family, so it was difficult to be stuck 1,500 miles away from everyone all the time. It's a good thing that I have some free nationwide minutes, otherwise my phone bill would have been crazy! One of the best weeks I had during that first year was when my entire family drove down from New Jersey to spend Thanksgiving with me. Aunts, uncles, cousins, and my immediate family drove through the night one Wednesday while I was on call at work. By morning time, they greeted me with warm smiles and good food on the stove. We stuffed our faces with turkey, candied yams, veggies, and delicious pecan pie. I was so happy, and we had a fabulous time laughing, shopping, and frolicking on the beach. Weekends like that helped me get through my intern year, and I suggest the same for other people far away from home and missing the love of their families.

Back to work. By the end of the year, things were looking up. It doesn't happen overnight, but with each day, each rotation, it all somehow becomes more manageable. You become friends with your fellow residents, and they become like a second family. You help save some lives, and feel good about the comfort you bring to patients' families. The need for studying never ends as a doctor, but before you know it, your rotations in Emergency Medicine, Pulmonology, Pediatrics, Cardiology, and the ICU are over. Your Transitional Year has come to an end, and next year, you're on to Anesthesia…

5:00 a.m. The alarm clock goes off and I jump out of bed. I rush off to the bathroom and get my shower going. A half hour later, I emerge (I gotta cut my showers down, I know!) and get dressed in pants and a nice shirt. I comb my hair, throw on my white coat, and snap my pager onto my outfit. I run downstairs and start my car in the garage. I pull out a granola bar from my pocket, and zoom off to the hospital. I arrive, look for a parking space, then run into the locker room. At our program, we have to arrive in professional attire (no sweats or scrubs), so our first stop is always the locker room to change. Next I head upstairs to put on a surgical hat, mask, and gloves, then go to 'the board' for a quick look. The board is a large dry erase board where all of our assignments for the day are listed. All of the surgeries taking place that day are either on the board or on a paper that you can carry around. I look on the board for my name, and see that I am scheduled to work in operating room #4 for the day. I rush off to room four and turn on the anesthesia machine. The machine automatically runs through a 15-minute check-out process, which I supervise. While this happens, I also draw up the medications I will use for my first case, lay out the vital sign monitors, and cue up the patient's medical record on the room's computer.

Once my room is all set up and ready for the operation to begin, I run to the holding area in order to meet the patient. I interview and examine him, get him to sign a consent form, start an intravenous line, discuss the case with my attending, and draw up more pain medication for potential use. After receiving word that the nurses in the OR are ready for us to begin, I wheel the patient back and start the process of putting him to sleep. I help him get onto the operating table and make him comfortable. I hook him up to the blood pressure, heart, and oxygen saturation monitors. I give him pre-medication drugs that will help him relax and will prevent infection. I place an oxygen mask over his face, hang fluids to keep him hydrated, begin my computer record, and let my attending know that I'm ready to officially begin. The attending arrives; I give the final medications to induce sleep. I manually give deep breaths of 100% oxygen; when he is completely relaxed and asleep, I pull out my endotracheal tube, bite block, suction machine, and Macintosh blade. I place a breathing tube down his throat successfully and hook him up to the anesthesia machine that will breathe for him while the surgery proceeds. I then clean up, make sure the patient is warm, administer the remaining medications, and fill in the missing information on my computer record. Now it's time to wait for the surgical team to arrive and make the first incision.

Over the next 2 hours, I monitor the patient's vitals, periodically give pain medicine and muscle relaxants, update the chart, record urine output, keep a steady supply of fluids going, and do everything to ensure that the patient makes it through the surgery without incident. As the surgeon closes the wound and walks out, I start letting the patient wake up. I let the muscle relaxants wear off (so he is no longer paralyzed), and let him start breathing on his own. With my attending by my side once again, I am able to remove the breathing tube, shut off the anesthesia machine, and wind up the case. I grab my paperwork and wheel the patient to our assigned spot in the recovery room. I hook him up to vital sign monitors again and give report to the recovery room nurse. I tell her all about the patient and the operation, and once I'm sure that he will recover okay, I leave him in her care. I return any unused pain medication, meet and interview my next patient, discuss the case with my attending, clean and restock the operating room, then wait for the next operation to get underway. This process continues several times through the day, with a 30-minute break for lunch somewhere along the way.

Around 5:00 p.m., the scheduled surgeries for the

day come to an end, and my call night begins. I'm on call once or twice per week, and must sleep in the hospital in order to take care of patients. I talk to the board-runner (the attending physician who is in charge of personnel assignments for the day) to find out where my services are needed. There is no planned surgery that I need to stay in the operating room for, so I go to the security office, get a call room key, then head to my room in the obstetrics wing of the hospital. I will be covering obstetric patients overnight, so I get sign-out from the resident who was taking care of obstetric patients during the day. Sign-out is where I hear about all of the post-delivery women, the epidurals that are currently in place, and the patients in danger of needing an emergency c-section or procedure overnight. I walk around the wing in order to meet all of the patients. I find out how they're doing, and note who is still in need of an epidural or close to delivery. I make sure that all paperwork is done, and place my pager number on the board for nurses to quickly contact me if needed. My next stop is the cafeteria to get dinner before things shut down for the night. With my armful of food, I retreat back to my call room and do one of several things. I may watch television, read/study, make phone calls, or get some hard-to-come-by sleep. Tonight, I choose to take a nap, and it's a good thing that I did, because I get a call about a laboring patient who now needs an epidural placed. The attending and I go to her room and go through the 30-minute process to get her comfortable. There is another patient who needs an epidural right after her, and later, in the middle of night, there is a c-section delivery of twins that we must perform.

On nights that we don't cover obstetric patients (nurse anesthetists can also cover them), we do overnight surgeries and take care of the orthopedic patients who have had painful operations to their knees, hips, and shoulders, along with any patients with acute and chronic pain issues. Other teams can be called in to handle heart surgeries, brain operations, or liver transplants, and if there is no other case for the resident to handle, he/she can assist with those massive undertakings. Not all nights are jam-packed with action, but there are some nights where that is the case. At 7:00 a.m., when there is a lull in the action, I sign-out to the team coming on duty, then either go to morning lecture (if there is one), or head home to rest until the next day.

The thing that upsets me about anesthesia – and just about the only thing – is the lack of respect we are given. People think we do nothing, know nothing, and are good for nothing. There is the perception that all we do is sit in the operating room drinking coffee and reading newspapers; that we are unnecessary members of the health care team that can be bossed around and undervalued. I am of the opinion that we are some of the smartest, calmest, and most skilled physicians out there. A good anesthesiologist can walk into any OR and take any patient through any procedure, big or small. You have to know about each type of surgery – which ones involve lots of blood loss, which ones are particularly painful in certain areas thus interfering with recovery, and which ones affect the autonomic nervous system thus causing lots of potentially dangerous physiological changes. We help women deliver babies safely and with minimal pain, we deal with pain patients who are at their wit's end and can't be helped by other doctors, and we man the Intensive Care Unit with the most complicated patients that others don't know how to handle. Anesthesiologists can take command during a code situation and will know exactly which drug to give or life-saving maneuver to perform in order to save a life. We deal with life and death every minute of every work day – our patients usually cannot breathe or communicate while we work with them, so we must listen to their bodies all the more closely and rely on our extensive medical knowledge to help them through. I'd like to see any other profession try that and do it with the flair and grace that we do. Emergency Room physicians come close to our proficiency in critical situations, but again, our job encompasses so much and is so important to so many types of patients.

Like I said, my days as a resident can be long and busy, or they can be routine and calm. I knew what I wanted from an early age, and as I go through each rotation, I cherish all of the knowledge handed down and yearn for the day when I'll 'know it all'. I love both busy days and calm ones because I love anesthesia, and my only hope is that everyone in medicine loves their jobs just as much. Wish me luck as I continue with my medical journey, and I wish you luck in finding something to satisfy and challenge you...

■ ■

I got to St. Luke's Hospital safely, parked in the physician lot, and stumbled toward the admitting area. I placed my small overnight bag on my lap and let the young clerk behind the desk know that I was there to be admitted. She made some quick phone calls and instructed me to take a seat. After a few minutes, an orderly arrived with a wheelchair and transported me up to the fourth floor. The process was very quick, since my doctor had called ahead to make all the admitting arrangements. I got to the room, put my things down, and listened to the nurse's 'new patient' spiel. I changed clothes, settled onto the bed, and called my parents. My mother was busy on the phone and internet scrambling to find a flight to Jacksonville that night for her and my father (man, she is good!). She had already arranged to take time off of work through the Family Medical Leave Act (FMLA), and was anxious to get to me and take care of me in whatever ways I needed her.

The neurology resident on call soon came to my room to take an in-depth history and do a thorough physical exam. We talked for almost an hour, and after I told him all about the occurrences of the last three weeks, he left the room to secure materials in order to perform a lumbar puncture (LP, or spinal tap) on me. He returned with a sterile tray full of needles and collecting tubes. He put on his sterile gloves and draped a sterile towel over my back. I lay motionless on my side near the edge of the bed while he numbed up my lower back with some Lidocaine. He then unsheathed a large gauge needle and stuck it in my back. He maneuvered it around and tried to inch it forward. We waited for a clear stream of cerebrospinal fluid (CSF) to flow from the needle, but it never came. After several long minutes of poking and lots of position changes, we concluded that our spinal tap attempt was not going to work. He apologized profusely, then left to call the Radiology department and schedule another attempt

44

under fluoroscopy (a special x-ray technique) for the next day.

I closed my eyes and let it all sink in. Things were moving very quickly. That morning I was working diligently in the ICU, and now I was a helpless patient, grasping for some simple answers. I have never been sick a day in my life, and have certainly never had these odd tests performed on me. No x-rays or ankle sprains – I've barely even needed antibiotics for the occasional chest cold. Needless to say, I was scared about all of these recent developments, but there was nothing I could do about it. Much later that evening, my parents arrived in Florida, and I dutifully filled them in on the afternoon's events. Because of the late hour, they decided to stay at my house until the morning, and so I bid them goodnight and settled into my lumpy hospital bed, happy to put this tumultuous day behind me.

At 4 a.m. I was awakened so that an orderly could record my vital signs. At 7 a.m. there were more vital signs and also some blood work done. My parents shuffled into my room at about 8 a.m., then we waited for the neurology team to enter and supply whatever answers they came across. They came at around 9, and I was thrilled to speak with their attending. He interviewed and examined me, but of course, he had no new answers to give. I had to wait until my lumbar puncture was completed, and who knew that it would take all day to get it done?! I was rolled down to Radiology, but spent forever waiting. I spoke to my boss and plenty of my colleagues while in the waiting area, and even took a couple of naps. Finally I was rolled into the room where the procedure would be performed. It was quick and painless, even a little exciting for a girl who likes blood & guts to see the needles and the collection process.

The next day, the neurology team visited again, this time with a plan of action in mind. They informed me that there was no evidence of brain infection, abscess, or tumor on my spinal tap results. There was no sign of meningitis, and my history didn't fit the pattern of some genetic rarity. They could not definitively diagnose me with anything at that time, but decided to put me on medication to decrease my symptoms. A 'wait and see' approach would be best to uncover if I was experiencing a one-time medical setback, or if I truly had a debilitating, chronic neurological disease. That night, I was given my first dose of steroids. I would be taking 1 gram of intravenous corticosteroids per day – not to be confused with anabolic steroids, the frequently abused steroids for enhanced physical performance and appearance. Along with those meds, I would have to take pills to prevent the ulcers, infections, depression, and increased blood sugar levels they could cause. I lost a little weight from the meds (contrary to what they normally cause), and noticed that my hair was growing out of control. During the day I worked with physical therapists to help me relearn how to walk. We worked on balance, strength, and coordination; soon I didn't need to hold onto walls in order to walk, but I couldn't turn my head too quickly without risking a fall. I ordered lots of food from the cafeteria and even cracked my books open a few times. I chatted with all the nurses who worked on my floor and enjoyed all of my co-worker visitors. After 6 days of this, it was time for me to go home. My IV steroid therapy was over, and I would continue my treatment and recovery at home. I felt a lot better about the situation – I knew that no matter what the final diagnosis was I would be fine. I actually looked forward to getting back to work and taking care of my health.

I did just that once I got home. My parents stayed with me, and my aunt, brother, and sister even came to visit during my downtime. I was confined to a blanket on the living room floor for the first few days since I couldn't climb the stairs easily to my bedroom. I tried to go the vegetarian route in an attempt to optimize my health (that didn't last long). I took short walks around my neighborhood to build strength. I got my wish to return to work after a month or so, because that's when I went back to anesthesia part-time. I did fairly well there, even though I required lots of supervision to ensure that no mistakes were made. I staffed the obstetrics floor during the day, and the next month moved on to the recovery room. Things were going great and I was eager to get back to the operating room that I loved. I got that wish the next month when I started my rotation providing anesthesia for patients undergoing orthopedic surgery procedures.

Nerves didn't deter me from doing a good job in the OR – I arrived extra early and double checked everything I did. I had no time for fooling around, and even shunned the extra help my fellow residents tried to offer. No matter that I spilled some powerful narcotics when mixing syringes in the mornings. It was a small, yet costly mistake. Who cares that I couldn't answer some of my attending's simple questions during cases. It's not that I was forgetting things, I must have been more focused on getting through the day's surgeries without a calamity. Yes, it was embarrassing when I passed out during an operation, but with some rest, I was back at it the next day. It was a fluke when I forgot to turn on the anesthesia machine after intubating a patient, right? Anyone could have made that possibly fatal error…right?? I really thought that I was just out of practice after being out of the OR for almost three months, but my program director was not of the same opinion. She noticed a big drop in my performance and didn't feel comfortable leaving patient lives in my hands when I was obviously having some problems. One day, I was yanked out of my operating room and sent down to employee health. Fearing that I still had some lingering health issues, I was evaluated again. I sat with doctors and psychotherapists, each probing into my psyche to find the root of the problem. I was scheduled for neuropsychiatric testing, which, to my surprise, showed impaired information processing and calculation time. My reaction time was slowed and my attention to detail was noticeably absent. I didn't seem to recognize my deficiencies, and that's a dangerous situation when dealing with patients. I was told to take more disability time off - just to allow more time to heal. Just to get back to normal.

So I took time off. I rested on my couch, and I visited friends and family. It was nice to slow down for once, but I had to go back to my neurologist when more numbness appeared in my hands a month later. This time, the entire right side of my body developed an uncomfortable pins-and-needles sensation. It wasn't painful, but I didn't want anyone or anything to touch my skin because it caused a very, very strange feeling – almost like my skin was burning. I hoped that it would go away on its own, but my doctor wouldn't let me get off that easily. I did yet another MRI and some more blood work. The medical team had long discussions and pored over all of the gathered information. They found additional MRI-identified brain lesions in several areas, and the 'pins-and-needles' episode didn't help my case. At my next office visit, they sat me down and were finally able to diagnose me with something: Multiple sclerosis (MS).

Multiple sclerosis, huh? So that's what it all came down to. That's what was causing such turmoil in my life. MS is a disease of myelin, the body's protective covering over nerves. Without myelin, signaling throughout the body is impaired, the autoimmune system attacks itself, and episodes of inflammation lead to varied clinical symptoms. The diagnosis came out of nowhere, since no one in my family has ever had any neurological diseases that I knew of. I didn't know what to think or how to feel. I was happy that I didn't 'feel' sick, and that I wasn't in any pain. I guess I could handle a few relapses here and there - my biggest question was about life expectancy. Would MS take years off of my life? Could I experience a severe exacerbation that would put me in a coma - or worse, in the grave? How long would it take before I was wheelchair bound and confined to my room? What could I do to perfect my health and prolong my healthy years? How much time did I have??

I started on daily medication and kept a small journal detailing my symptoms. I answered questions from family members whenever they called to check on my progress. At first I felt ok with this news. I had researched MS, guillain-barre syndrome, lyme disease, and other similar sicknesses when all of this started. I kinda knew that MS (or something like it) was coming, so I accepted the diagnosis when it was handed down and looked ahead to the next step. It was a real pain giving myself those injections all the time, but it had to be done. I would fall over while trying to jab my thigh with those tiny medication needles, but like I said, it had to be done. I started experiencing more and more fatigue – it got to a point where I couldn't sleep at night, but couldn't keep my eyes open during the day. I avoided strenuous activities, as I would experience setbacks whenever I inadvertently did too much. My right leg would get very tight and heavy if I was on it for too long. If you looked closely, you would see me limping around whenever I tried to walk. I ate well (sort of) and tried to rest often. Again, I thought that with these new medications and more time to heal, I would be back on my feet in no time.

I am unhappy to report, however, that a few medication adjustments and symptom exacerbations later, I am *still* out of work on long-term disability, trying to find my way. No miraculous recoveries for me. No return to my pre-MS state. I can only sit on the couch and pass the time with game shows on t.v. and web-surfing on the internet. I am watching my anesthesia colleagues finish up their time in residency while I sit on the sidelines, desperately eager to get back into the game. I am living life as a defenseless patient, and not as the proud caretaker I once was. I am fighting with insurance companies and claim specialists, trying to prove that I really am sick and unable to work. I am losing faith in the resiliency of my young body, but hopefully not in the potential that I still possess as a young, capable, and motivated doctor.

I honestly don't know what I'm going to do. I try to exercise when I can, but my symptoms often make that difficult. Extreme fatigue, heart palpitations, weakness, headaches, and poor balance prevent me from doing too much physical activity. I can't drive for fear of another double vision attack, making it impossible to see the road and avoid oncoming traffic. I try to keep up with my studies and do some daily reading, but again, my symptoms make it hard. It's no small task to read a textbook when your eyes hurt from the constant fatigue. I can barely do anything academic when I forget ideas mid-sentence and can't find the simple everyday words to express my thoughts.

I am now thinking that I will have to switch gears and find something else to do in the realm of medicine. Maybe I'll work for a community service group, an advocacy team, a non-profit organization, or a research firm. Maybe a pharmaceutical company will have me and I can work on a cure for multiple sclerosis or other devastating diseases. Maybe I'll travel one day and do great things in remote, neglected areas across the globe. Maybe I'll go back to school and get that public health degree that was so appealing to me as a new medical student. I don't know what's in store for me, or what I should be doing in my downtime. Right now though, I am following doctor's orders, and am taking it easy. I appreciate everyone's concern for me, but I honestly resent their inability to leave me alone with my thoughts on the situation. Family and friends are constantly trying to get me to *do* things – regardless of how many times I remind them of my present physical state. They want me back to work even more than *I* do, and it's getting old having to explain things over and over again. I can seriously entertain those thoughts of medical greatness only if I ever regain the physical or mental stamina to do so. At this moment, I simply have to reflect on the ups and downs of the past year and gear up for the next inning. I have to rethink things, reorganize, and prioritize. I have to see where God takes me, and have faith that it will all work out for the best.

I don't say all of this to depress anyone. I don't want to discourage anyone from following their passion. Remember that I loved my job – my journey, my life. I accomplished the things that I dreamed of doing as a child, and touched the lives of many. I just wish that I had more to tell you about my time in residency, as short as it was. I wish that this break came as a result of careful consideration and deliberate planning, and not because of some unforeseen health scare. I don't know what is going to happen in my life, but I do know that I'll land on something bigger and better someday soon, and will be a better person for having gone through this ordeal. I know that my life will go on, and that the good things in store for me will still find a way to my doorstep. This is just a small hiccup in my journey – a time to step back, switch gears, and find a way to make this situation work.

I want everyone reading this to find and nurture *their* passion, and do everything in their power to make their dreams become reality. I want all aspiring doctors to enjoy the ride, learn as much as possible, be good to your patients, and be great to yourself. Never stop searching for the answers or become jaded by the ills that may surround you. Never compromise your morals or forget the Hippocratic oath that comes with your medical degree. We can do without the people who aren't serious about medicine – those only out for a buck, and those who can't be bothered with an honest day's work. Keep grounded and keep in touch with the teachers, friends, family, and classmates that helped you along the way. Keep that compassion alive, and find ways to be better everyday. Keep me in your prayers, and when you win that Nobel Prize or find that cure for cancer, reach back to help the students coming behind you, eager to make their mark and do their part. You've already made the decision to become a part of the medical field, now make the decision to be great and do great things. I know, without the smallest doubt, that you can do it - just like this girl from a small town with a small health problem did. Good luck!

ADDENDUM

I ended my chapter with some sad news, but that's how life is. Things happen and sometimes you are flung into situations you never imagined. True to my word, though, things are starting to look up for me. I have been out on disability for over 2 years, and have made some medication switches along the way. I now have a little more energy, and my strength is making a modest comeback!

I was surprised by a job offer recently - my medical school (the wonderful NJMS) expressed some interest in hiring me for an administrative position!! This would be perfect for me, since I would get to work in the field of medicine, I wouldn't have to deal with the fast pace of residency, and I would be helping the students and communities that I've always had a passion for giving back to.

I view this as an example of how remaining faithful and positive can help any situation. I have never given up on myself and will not let this medical misfortune ruin my life. It's still too early to know what will happen with that job position or my overall health, but all will be well – I just know it!!

CAREER SNAPSHOT

IN FOCUS: ANESTHESIOLOGY

Years in graduate school: 4 years medical school

Years in post-graduate training: 4 years residency

Fellowship: Critical care medicine, pain management, regional anesthesia, etc.

Salary: average annual salary ranges from $300,000 to $450,000 and up

Pros: flexible schedule, high salary, varied cases and procedures to perform

Cons: in-hospital call often required, high liability/malpractice insurance rates

Extra info: number of anesthesiologists completing fellowship is approximately 30%

Information taken from http://www.aamc.org/cim

"Finding Yourself In Medicine"

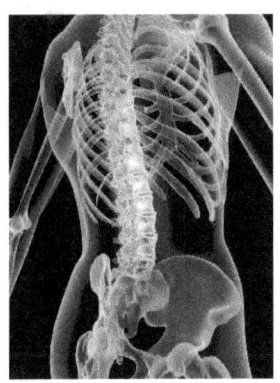

Miguel A. Coba, M.D.
PGY-3, Department of Physical Medicine and Rehabilitation
University of Medicine and Dentistry of New Jersey
New Jersey Medical School
Newark, NJ

IN THIS CHAPTER...

* What does PM&R mean? What can that type of doctor do?

* How is a PM&R residency program structured?

* What fellowships can a PM&R doctor do?

* How does one make the decision to go into medicine?

* Does religion have any place in medicine?

What is it about medicine that attracted you? How did you know that you wanted to spend your life doing it?

From an early age, I knew that I liked science, particularly physics and math. My father was a doctor, so I figured that I could make my parents happy while doing something in the sciences. I was thinking about engineering, but since I wasn't the greatest, most hard working high school student, I didn't think I would actually achieve anything big in life. I saw myself working in a lab or something – and that was good enough for me. But lo and behold, I guess life had other plans for me. I ended up majoring in biology with a focus in pre-med in college. And it turned out that I did really well. I didn't find things to be too difficult for me, so I excelled in my studies. I don't know why exactly, I guess because school was more exam oriented – less floating around trying to learn about everything like in high school. Things were more a bit more focused and structured. Plus, I went into a pre med program, so I had counselors along the way to tell me what to do. Everything was laid out and I didn't have to do much extra work to figure things out. I never really got the chance to try other things in depth, but I was happy that the thing I went in for is the thing I graduated with. Everybody told me the hard work would come in medical school, but my college experience wasn't the most awe-inspiring thing. Just following a path and doing what I had to do.

How was medical school for you?

It was fun. The best four years of my life. I enjoyed it more than college because I got to drink

(I was finally of age!). No, seriously - it was a lot more focused in the sense that all you have to do is go study and not worry about other subjects, random people, or classes. I know a lot of people get very stressed out and others think that doctors are supposed to be the best and achieve above all else, but I'm not that type of person. I'm very laid back – don't get me wrong – I do stress, especially during exams, but not like the others who can go a whole year and never relax, do anything fun, or give themselves a break. So because I was able to handle the workload and the potentially stressful environment, yeah it was a lot of fun. I got to meet a lot of great people.

What was the hardest part of medical school? Was it a class? A professor? A particular subject or exam? What are some of the tough things you dealt with?

Failure, maybe. I went through 4 years of college being at the top of my class, and then there was the rude awakening of medical school where things are harder and classes require more focus. For the first time in a long time, I had to adjust my studying and outlook - so that was a tough adjustment for me. Luckily I dealt with the failure and learned from my mistakes.

Also learning to deal with patients, attendings, and the rest of the health care team was difficult. I think I had a hard time when we began our clinical rotations, because for the first time I had to get acclimated to being in the spotlight during rounds and giving presentations almost every day. I am a naturally shy and quiet person in certain situations, so I don't often say anything or volunteer answers. I've gotten better - more comfortable with the way things work - but it certainly wasn't easy at first.

Did you ever regret going into medicine?

It's not that I necessarily regret going into medicine, but everyone has those hard days where they wonder if they should have gone into something else. There's a lot of complaining about your day, and I definitely have those times when I think, "oh – I should have picked an easier career", but that doesn't really matter or help things in the long run.

Why did you go into PM&R?

I liked Physical Medicine and Rehabilitation for different reasons. I liked the anatomy involved – that was one of my favorite classes in medical school. Even after that class though, I still wasn't sure that I was going to do PM&R – I thought for a while I would go into general surgery or trauma surgery. Turns out that they really weren't the right choice for someone as laid back as I am. When I did my third year surgery rotations, it was confirmed that I couldn't spend the rest of my life in that kind of hostile, competitive environment. The impression I got was that it was abusive towards residents. I worked with some really great surgeons but it wasn't enough to sway me into that specialty. I also did medicine rotations but never really liked it. My sister and brother-in-law are doctors, so I got plenty of exposure to their fields as well. Even with all of that exposure, I never developed a passion for *any* of the other specialties out there.

I knew that I liked anatomy, I knew I wanted something with a lot of patient interaction, and I knew that I wanted hands-on work on a daily basis. I knew about PM&R kind of early because at our medical school we were exposed to things early in our studies. Plus, PM&R had the reputation of being very chill, so I liked that aspect of it. It's not as chill as people make it out to be, but it definitely is better than some other fields. So with all of that in mind, I went for it. During my PM&R rotation, I worked with two great attendings, and they taught me things that we didn't even learn in med school pathology or anatomy classes. I learned in depth things that got me even more interested in the field. These attendings knew about everything, and that intellectual excellence attracted me even more to PM&R. In one week, I would see a few patients in the outpatient clinic, but even that was a level beyond what I had known, and more than a textbook would have ever shown me. They sent me to Kessler, our rehabilitation center, and I saw patients in a whole new light. I had seen similar patients at other hospitals – those on the brink of death in situations that seemed hopeless. But at Kessler, I saw them receive innovative treatments and recover to a level I didn't think they could get to. I thought, 'wow - if I can be a part of this, that would be awesome'. Then I did more rotations, and it all confirmed that I was headed in the right direction.

What does your job entail now? What are you responsible for? What rotations do you do?

PM&R, or physiatry, is split into several different aspects. The easiest way to split it is into the outpatient/musculoskeletal doctors and the inpatient/rehabilitation doctors. So our rotations are kind of split that way (with the addition of pediatric rotations). Outpatient rotations include clinics at different hospitals. Here, you see general musculoskeletal complaints: chronic pain, professional athletes and their physical issues, shoulder/back/knee pain, arthritis, and tendonitis. You can diagnose peripheral neuropathies and central nervous system disorders with nerve conduction studies and other electrodiagnostic modalities. Inpatient rotations are where you deal with rehab patients, stroke patients, amputee care, prosthetics, orthotics, and pain management.

Call is generally 2-6 times per month for us, and it is taken by one resident. Our attendings remain at home, because rehab patients should be close to medically stable and there shouldn't be many random admissions overnight. We may have planned overnight admissions – but only if the patient arrives after hours. We get called about very different things in the hospital and often need to see patients in the emergency room. There is no real overnight call during outpatient rotations - some sites may have home call until 10pm. Those hospitals (like the VA hospital) have medical coverage overnight where other medical residents take care of fevers or other small issues that come up with our patients while we are away at night. Then, in the morning, we tell our attending about what happened with all of the PM&R patients and go home. There is no large team of health care professionals like on medicine wards, and no need to round each morning – our attending will round alone on his/her patients. Rehab has no continuity of care issues in the traditional sense since almost every rotation is one on one with the attending. That's a real difference from internal medicine teams, but it allows for great teaching and hands-on experience.

What do you like most about residency, about your experience in PM&R?

Well I don't really like the musculoskeletal side of PM&R. I can't deal with the patients who just complain about their shoulder all day long. I know they have legitimate complaints, but I don't get fulfillment from handling those cases. I like spinal cord cases and total brain injury. As much as we know about anatomy and special advanced tests, sometimes we still don't know what's going on. There is no routine component to it, and every case is vastly different. We don't do a lot of 'cookbook medicine' - where you throw every test or therapeutic option at a patient and hope something sticks. Here, you get to experiment and really think through cases.

From the outside, you may think it's as easy as 'I'm paralyzed from the waist or neck down, and that's it', but it's so much more complicated than that. The whole physiology of the body changes – the patient's way of life changes and problems that didn't exist before now have to be considered. The amount of research being done is enormous, the field is constantly evolving, and the relationship you can build with patients is very rewarding. Also, I like that I have a lot of time to deal with family and friends. All in all, residency has been a wonderful experience for me.

What's the worst thing about it?

Being limited in what you can do. Say, for instance, we are doing injections or some type of therapy on a patient, but find lots of other problems unrelated to their musculoskeletal complaints. Psychosocial issues may come up – things that a patient would benefit from if they were addressed and corrected, like caretaker access, or mental health care. However, the way the system is now, you can't go into the patients psych history on the computer, and Medicare won't allow you to spend the extra 10 minutes probing the issue. That is extremely frustrating and I wish there were a way to deliver more complete care.

What has surprised you about residency?

How not hard it is. How I can get away with things. Sometimes I go a long time without picking up a book and attendings still think I'm smart! I always say, 'if u only knew'…It's a great feeling to accomplish difficult things easily and conquer the fears that you started with. I was very nervous when beginning residency, but I am receiving great training and can handle any future surprises that come my way.

How well prepared were you for residency? How did you get past it?

I wasn't prepared at all. Medical school doesn't quite prepare you for residency. It's another world entirely, and I felt lost. I didn't know anything. I knew books, but not real clinical patient stuff. Patients don't present the way you encounter them on the USMLE. They don't walk into your office and say, 'I have nasal congestion, malaise, and hyperthermia". All they say is, 'I don't feel well', and you then have to investigate the problem.

The dynamics of it all - having to deal with other residents and specialties was also tough during the adjustment to residency. You're trying to take care of your patients, but so many things can stand in your way. I've realized that you just have to do it. There's no way around the adjustment. You deal and adjust, and little by little it becomes more comfortable. Soon after starting residency, you can combine your book knowledge with the people skills and leadership that you pick up along the way.

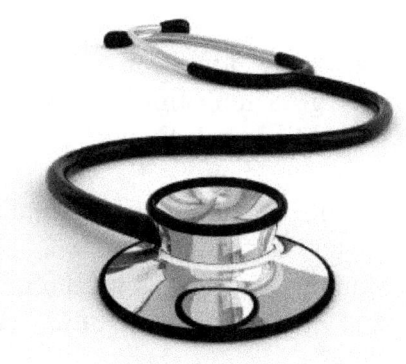

What do you want to do next? What comes after residency?
What are your options?

I'm going to do a fellowship in spinal cord. After that – I'll go wherever God takes me. Ideally I would like to do something where I can see the whole gamut from acute injury in a hospital setting, to acute rehabilitation, to recovery, to discharge, and then follow up as an outpatient for years down the road. I'd love to do something to incorporate all of that but I may be dreaming there. It is possible and some people do it, but that's not the typical job in my field. The big thing in my field now is that people, especially in the top tier programs, want to do outpatient procedures - like pain medicine maneuvers.

I think I have a skewed perspective when it comes to fellowships and jobs, because I'm in one of the best PM&R residency programs. That will open up a lot of doors for me, and it won't be too hard to find a good job when I'm ready. PM&R isn't like dermatology with the competition – we can pretty much get jobs anywhere.

Is time management a problem for you?

Yeah. I don't have time to do all the things I would like to, but I think that's life. I do all the important things, but I would love to do *everything* - read all the books, do all the fun stuff with friends, be a good spouse, son, and brother, do research, etc. The perfectionist in all of us would probably like to do the same, but the reality is that we only get 24 hours in a day, and we need to eat & sleep once in awhile. I think I manage my time well – I just wish I had more of it!

As a physiatrist, you must see some pretty traumatic injuries - how does spirituality play into your job? How does it affect it, if at all?

I think my job affects me, but my religion really helps me deal with life in general. If I see a really sad story (which I see a lot), I realize that I have a different view of human suffering. What most people see as tragic, I guess I don't. For instance, there was a patient that came in with a necrotic toe, and was soon intubated after suffering a stroke. He had surgery for the toe, but his graft didn't take, and he will lose the limb anyway. He will have significant deficits for the rest of his life, and we have to work with him to piece his life back together. In this case, I don't see his situation as being the end of the world. Not to sound non-empathetic, but I think that things happen for a reason. I believe in God and His love for us all, so just because something bad happens, it doesn't mean that the love disappears. It could turn out to be the best thing to happen for a person someday. That's how I see things. We all suffer in life, but that suffering has brought me closer to God and taught me certain things about myself. I appreciate all of the miracles in my life and the lives of those around me. I don't know what kind of resident or doctor I would be without my spirituality to guide me, so I am very thankful for it.

What do you wish someone told you about medicine before you started medical school? Any last minute advice to share?

I wish that someone insisted that I knew what I was getting into. Every student should know that medicine is not an easy thing, and that hard work is the name of the game. Many people become disillusioned and say, 'I hate my job – if only I knew...' That may be personality related, meaning that those people would be miserable in *any* field, but it really isn't that bad with self-reflection beforehand and perseverance throughout. If you understand the things you do and the reasons behind it, the journey to an M.D. might be a little easier. Be honest with yourself, even if you go into medicine for the "wrong" reasons like money or fame. If you think that'll make you happy, then own up to it, try it out, and stick with it. Above all else, be good to your patients, and never feel like you're stuck in a position or a field that isn't right for you.

CAREER SNAPSHOT

IN FOCUS: PHYSICAL MEDICINE AND REHABILITATION

Years in graduate school: 4 years medical school

Years in post-graduate training: 4 years residency

Fellowship: sports medicine, neuromuscular medicine, hospice/palliative medicine, etc.

Salary: average annual salary ranges from $140,000 to $260,000 and up

Pros: wide range of patient types and diseases treated, desirable schedule

Cons: deals with devastating medical events and difficult Rehabilitation

Extra info: this specialty is also known as Physiatry (fizz-EYE-uh-tree)

Information taken from http://www.aamc.org/cim

"You're Not A Real Doctor!"

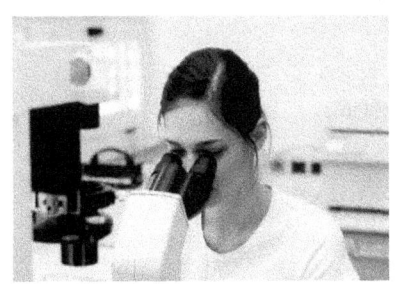

Yvelisse N. Suarez, M.D.
PGY-3, Department of Pathology
Mount Sinai School of Medicine, New York, NY

IN THIS CHAPTER...

* Why do people go into Pathology? What is the appeal?

* How much research is needed in the decision for residency?

* How should one approach the interview?

* What rotations do Pathology residents do?

* What options exist once residency is over?

The Birth of an Academic Doctor

I am currently a third-year Pathology resident who has no doubt that I made the right decision to go into pathology. In all honesty, though, the decision to enter Pathology was a rather difficult one. I entered medical school to be on the forefront of providing quality care for underprivileged communities. I am a Puerto Rican, who although I cannot speak perfect Spanish, can still communicate and get my point across. Of the 16,000+ medical students that graduate in a year, a mere 300 are Puerto Ricans. I naturally felt a social obligation to serve my community and thought it would be a crime if I used my education to be in front of a microscope instead of patients. I resisted the call of Pathology and during my clinical rotations as a third-year; I tried to decide between Surgery and Geriatrics for a specialty. I figured it would be great if I could work in an underserved community as a Spanish-speaking surgeon or if I took care of someone's *abuelita*. I did well on my clinical rotations, and my extracurricular activities and even my medical school were patient centered. Furthermore, I truly enjoyed seeing patients and connected with the personal side of human affliction which only added to my career conflict.

There was a slight problem however; I just could not see myself being happy for the next 40 years of my professional life if I did Surgery or Geriatrics. As much as I loved patients, there is a reality of clinical medicine that is quite ugly. In order to get compensated by insurance companies, there is pressure to see as many patients as possible which could compromise the way I envisioned practicing medicine. Being a doctor can be such as thankless profession; you can sacrifice your weekends, holidays, personal time, and at times your own health just to be rewarded with a lawsuit! We live in such a litigious society; I've seen many competent, caring doctors being sued for superfluous reasons so that some lawyer who only went to three years of graduate school can make a quick buck.

In addition, there is also the component of human error. I wondered how I would feel if I ever made an honest mistake that led to morbidity or demise of a patient. I am one of those people that actually feel bad when I accidentally step on an ant; I cannot imagine the feeling of harming someone after I've dedicated years of my life studying and training in order to take care of patients. But the truth is that it happens all the time, even to the smartest, most seasoned doctors in the hospital. With pathology, there is still that possibility of missing that metastatic focus or misdiagnosing a specimen which can adversely affect a patient but it is not actively harming a patient. Another thing I considered was how I would feel 20 years down the road as a surgeon or geriatrician? Would I still be excited about appendectomies or checking someone's blood pressure? Unfortunately, I thought the answer was no.

Early in my fourth year, I took the Surgical Pathology elective and was fascinated witnessing pathologists resemble "talking textbooks" whenever clinicians from various disciplines consulted them for answers. I respected the impact they had on patients' prognosis by arming clinicians with accurate diagnoses. Additionally, I realized that performing autopsies allows one to be an advocate for the deceased by using knowledge obtained to address causes of death and prevent future mortalities. To be certain pathology was my calling, I took fourth-year electives in Medicine and Surgery which only confirmed there was no other specialty I wanted to devote my life to. As far as not having patient interaction, I felt I could battle human affliction on a broader scale by influencing the daily care and management of patients using laboratory medicine. There is a misconception that pathologist don't have live patients so aren't real doctors. The truth is, most of the specimens we receive come from live patients which are depending on us to accurately diagnosis their disease so they can receive the proper treatment or follow-up.

One of the pathology attendings also told me I had "the eye" and would make an excellent pathologist. I noticed I preferred viewing a piece of tissue through a microscope as it provides more insight into a patient's disease than performing a complete history and physical exam. My interpersonal skills may not be used on patients and their families, but will be invaluable in building rapport and facilitating collaborations with colleagues. I felt the pathologists were the happiest doctors in the hospital and were the ones with the answers. They had no qualms about entering the field and were still excited about going into work even 30 years into practice. When I thought about it, it all just made sense.

Once I made the decision to go into pathology, it was application time. I applied to the east coast programs from Boston to Miami. I was assured that since I was an American graduate, I would have no problems getting my first choice. In pathology, there are many spots available however, getting into a top competitive program with good fellowship options is not that easy, even as an American graduate. The applicant pool is actually getting more competitive as medical students are starting to realize what Pathology has to offer. The board scores and class ranks are getting higher, less foreign graduates are getting spots, and medical students with multiple publications are becoming standard. You don't need a Ph. D. to get into Pathology but it is highly attractive and some research-oriented programs actually have most of their residents with Ph.D.'s. Thank God I got into Pathology when I did!

The Interview

Interviews for pathology are usually low stress, friendly, and tend to last the whole day. You will get interviewed by several attendings, have a tour of the facilities and usually there is a lunch with current residents. The lunch is one of the most important parts of the interviewing process because this is when you get real feel of a program. Be prepared to ask the following questions:

- How is the autopsy rotation/responsibilities organized i.e. are you pulled from rotations to do an autopsy? Is there a diener (a morgue attendant, responsible for handling, moving, and cleaning a corpse)? How many autopsies are done in a year and do residents have to share cases?

- Is there protected didactic time?

- How much time are you given to preview the slides?

- What is the surgical volume? What is the diversity of the specimens?

- Do you sign out everything you gross?

- Do fellows interfere with your training?

- What are the responsibilities during anatomical pathology call? How often is it?

- What are the responsibilities during clinical pathology call? And how often is it?

- Do you take call from home? Are there call rooms?

- Are there outside rotations? How do you get to them and far are they from the main hospital?

- How accommodating is the program, if you wanted to switch from AP/CP to AP only or CP only and vice versa?

- Is there a book and/or conference fund for residents?

- Are most residents single or married? Do residents have any social events together?

- Where have residents gone for fellowship?

I said most interviews were low stress, however, I did encounter one unpleasant program. The atmosphere of this Ivy League, New York City program seemed stuffy and cold. At the end of the interview day, the Director actually went through my grades and asked me to explain what happened in the courses that I did not "Honor"! Basically, every line of my application of was questioned and to top it off, the Director pointed out how inferior my application was compared to other applicants! If that was the case, why did they feel the need to waste my time? And toll money? They didn't need to offer me an interview if they thought I was so inferior. This is a rare occurrence in Pathology and there is a rumor this Director has left the program. Needless to say, I felt like I wasn't a good fit for the program.

Pathology programs, like most specialties are looking for residents that would mesh with the current residents and attendings. Despite what you might hear about pathologists being anti-social or weird, personality actually plays a big part in choosing residents. Unlike most specialties, the resident is face to face for hours with an attending while signing out, so programs want to be sure they can interact with you and that you are not too weird. Also, Pathology residency programs tend to be smaller than programs in medicine or surgery, so choosing residents who fit in and are dependable is more of an issue.

It was actually during these interviews that I found out more about pathology. Embarrassing to admit, but true. I think most people are familiar with anatomical pathology: biopsies, autopsies, and resections. Most medical students, including myself, have limited exposure to clinical pathology. This is the branch of pathology that deals with laboratory methods including microbiology, chemistry, and genetic testing.

I never really thought of who in the hospital oversees the CBCs, urinalyses, and type & cross tests that are regularly ordered. Apparently it is the pathologist that does everything behind the scenes. Basically, if there is anything in medicine that you don't know who is responsible for it, chances are, it is a pathologist. To my surprise, I was unaware that in some rotations such as blood banking and cytology, I would still need a stethoscope because I would see patients! Imagine that! The perfect combination, I would be able to see slides AND patients!

In selecting where I wanted to go, I looked at programs that would offer a large volume of specimens and had a good name. During medical school, I lived 20 minutes away from Manhattan and loved it, so I didn't envision myself content in a small town. For as long as I could remember, I always wanted to end up in New York City but I had always lived in the New York/New Jersey area so, I felt residency would be my opportunity to get to know a different city. I ranked programs in Boston highest because not only were they great programs but they were also located in a city. I then ranked programs in New York City; I interviewed at a few programs and liked most of them. When I interviewed at my program (Mount Sinai), I actually did like the comfortable atmosphere, felt like I belonged, and thought the residents were the coolest ones in the city. Don't forget that your fellow residents are going to have an impact on the next four years of your life so being able to get along with them and depend on them for support is important. I was however, terrified of the amount of work and hours the residents had. The advantage though, would be that there was an incredible exposure to a diverse pool of specimens and residents graduate prepared for anything that comes their way. The truth is that as a resident you want to be exposed to everything because you don't want to see things for the first time as an attending when all the responsibility is all on you. Also when you have a tough residency, fellowship is just that much easier. In the end, I decided this was the best New York City program for me.

Match Day

Match day came with a big surprise. As an American graduate, I thought I would get my first or second choice which was in Boston. I was mentally prepared for Boston and actually started looking on line for housing. I opened up the envelope and surprise! I was going to New York! For a split second, I was really disappointed but then I saw how relieved my mother was when she knew her daughter was going to stay in the area. Here I was just thinking about myself and my career while my family was scared I would match in Boston and move away from them. My Mother was joyous, couldn't stop hugging me, and was just full of tears. Ooops, sorry ma! I know the Match process is computerized and follows an algorithm but I also truly feel like there is a little divine intervention involved. No matter where you are placed, there is a reason for it even if it is unknown to you.

Great you matched! Now what?

It's time to celebrate! Enjoy your medical school friends while you can because everyone is going to move away and/or always be on call. Actually, being away from my medical school friends was a big transition for me. I went from studying several hours a day, everyday with my friends and then once medical school was over, there was nothing. My med school class had approximately 170 students so there was always someone around who wanted to study or blow off steam after exams; then I went into residency and there were only 6 people in my class and half were married! I still miss my medical school class so I suggest that you go to all the graduation parties that you can and, if at all possible, travel! The time period between graduation and July 1 goes by quickly so I took that time to look for housing on Craig's List, move in, unpack, and get acquainted with the city. The problem I encountered during this time was lack of funds. Loan money covers you until May and then if you are supposed to start on July 1st, you might not get a paycheck until the middle of July! In the meantime, I had to pay for June and July rent and a security deposit! We are talking about New York so this was actually thousands of dollars and doesn't include utilities or food! I ended up having to take a Medex loan and will worry about paying for it when I am an attending.

Residency Begins!

Before you start at any hospital, there is a basic orientation we are you get computer access, IDs, and the house staff manual. Orientation can start anywhere from mid-June until July 1st, so figure that in before you plan any vacations! Your pathology department will also have its own orientation. At my program, it was one day and I was totally overwhelmed by the amount of information I received. The next day, I started my first rotation which was surgical pathology at an outside institution.

My First Rotation

Most programs start their first-years in autopsy or they shadow an upperclassman. In my year, the program was trying something new and split the first year class into different rotations. I was not only lucky enough to start with surgical pathology but also at an outside hospital. On my first day, the chief tried to teach me how to gross. What an experience! I did not even know how to hold the tissue properly with forceps or how to take off the scalpel blade without injuring myself. Everything was new and everything had to be taught including how to make cassettes, how to ink, and even how to measure. I never felt so dumb and incompetent. I wish I had spent some time reading *Lester's Manual of Surgical Pathology* during the summer. Before starting residency, I had asked if there is anything I could do to prepare myself and everyone said I was going to pathology and didn't need to worry. Not true. If I could do it over again, I would have familiarized myself with how to dictate and would have learned the vocabulary I would need to intelligently describe a specimen. It was frustrating because I was so comfortable and adept at things I learned how to do in medical school like putting in IV lines and doing a complete history and physical; but then I started my residency absolutely clueless! Learning how to gross was a humbling experience.

In the beginning, everything in my dictations was just a tan mass and I was extremely slow because I just didn't know what to say. I included unnecessary descriptions and omitted important information. On top of that, there is also the actual physical grossing of the specimen which you could absolutely ruin if it's not done properly. I had training with the chief for two days and then I was left by myself. Luckily, the attendings were understanding and were always available for questions. This was a community hospital so I encountered diseases in an advanced state and anything that came out of the human body for the day came to me. So I mean EVERYTHING including flashlights and candles extracted from various orifices of the body. Great, another thing I didn't know about pathology!

Eventually, my grossing improved and dictations started to roll off my tongue. In my first month, I showed every big specimen to an attending, went over the proper way to gross it, and in the end, I actually didn't receive any complaints! Not too bad after all.

Molecular Pathology

My next rotation was Molecular Pathology which is the field of pathology that is constantly expanding and changing the practice of medicine. As pathologists, we are responsible for developing molecular assays, applying them to routine clinical use and overseeing their continued use. Our diagnostic laboratory tests genetic disorders such as prothrombin G20210A mutations, and Factor V Leiden. I spent this rotation reading standard operating procedures and familiarized myself with the basics of PCR (polymerase chain reaction), DNA, and reviewing my genetic disorders.

Autopsy

One of the reasons I entered pathology, was for the possibility of becoming a forensic pathologist. I have always been a fan of forensics and used to read forensic books as a high school student. In medical school, I witnessed a resident performing in autopsy and it didn't look too bad. I was looking forward to the rotation but unfortunately, I had it in October. I was the last of my classmates to have the rotation so I felt dumb...again.

At my program, there are two to three residents assigned to the autopsy rotation. Autopsies are performed seven days a week, 365 days a year, so we take call on the weeknight and weekends. If there are two people on autopsy, then there is a resident assigned to the pediatric rotation. When there are 3 people on autopsy, the residents are responsible for pediatric duties, which include placentas, products of conception, and fetal autopsies.

In my first month, there were 3 of us, so we rotated the pediatric duties and autopsies. The first two autopsy cases were done by the other two residents and when it came to my turn, they both took me through the autopsy. My first case was a 90-year-old female - a LOL, which in pathology means little old lady. We ended up finding an empyema, which was unexpected, and an incidental oncocytoma. The case itself wasn't difficult, but I immediately lost all interest in doing a fellowship in Forensic Pathology. There is something about feeling warm organs and the smells that turned me off. In addition, I did surgical pathology first and got used to the fast pace of grossing and signing out; autopsies just took too long. Most of the organs in a lot of the cases are free of pathology, so I didn't like having to gross normal organs. In addition to performing the actual autopsy which can take several hours, there is all the paperwork that has to be done. Prior to doing an autopsy, we usually go through the medical chart and speak to the clinician. After the autopsy, we have to document external findings which include every catheter, scar, and bruise; we describe internal findings; and write a microscopic description of our histological findings. Once that is done we do a clinicopathological correlate where we combine all the clinical and pathological findings, state the cause of death and contributing factors, and find supporting references. It can be a long process but it is one of the rotations where the things we learned during our clinical rotations in medical school are needed to uncover the cause of death.

In order to be eligible to sit for the boards, residents need to complete 50 autopsies and be the primary resident on at least 40 of them. Start logging your autopsies to the ACGME website as soon as you are done with an autopsy. The website doesn't ask for the primary diagnosis but do yourself a favor and enter it within the notes section because when it comes to apply for the boards in your fourth-year, you will need it to compile your list of autopsies complete with age, sex, date the autopsy was done, and primary diagnosis.

Microbiology

One of my favorite courses in medical school was microbiology so I was thrilled to have it in residency. During this rotation, residents rotate through different stations of the laboratory including bacteriology, mycology, parasitology, and virology. For our boards, we need to know how bacteria look on plates, the medium that certain organisms require to grow, how certain organisms are stained, and of course, their pathogenicity. For fungi, we need to know how they look on both sides of the plate, how they look when grown at different temperatures, and how they look under microscope. Honestly, one of my favorite stations is the parasitology lab because there is always some tick, worm, or eggs to look at. Microbiology is currently evolving and starting to use molecular diagnostics methods to identify HIV, HSV,

HCV, and HPV. Bacterial and mycobacterial identification by amplification and sequencing are performed and its uses will continue to grow in the future.

Pediatrics

The pediatric rotation was one of the more emotional rotations for me. In this rotation we do products of conception and come face to face with life and choice issues. One of the things that was particularly hard about this rotation was seeing perfectly normal fetuses being aborted while fetuses that were wanted were spontaneously aborted; it is heart-breaking to see a G4 P0 with another loss when you know how many times she has tried to conceive. My first pediatric autopsy was on a 30-week-old fetus that suddenly died in utero. The 40-year-old G2P0 mother had routine prenatal care and the day before had a normal ultrasound. She stopped feeling fetal movements, went to the hospital, and was found to have a fetal demise. At autopsy we found the umbilical cord wrapped twice, tightly around the fetus' neck.

One of my products of conception was difficult to do because she had such in an adorable face. Unfortunately, she also had amniotic band syndrome which destroyed her fingers bilaterally and disfigured her left arm. In general, pediatrics is a difficult rotation because it is so unpleasant to see dead babies. The positive that I was able to draw from this rotation is that when I perform an autopsy, I am able to help the family cope with their loss and provide the mother with a possible answer as to why she was unable to bring her baby home.

Gynecology

This is one of the busy rotations at our program because we gross and sign out everyday. The specimens that are done here include oncological resections, biopsies, and products of conception under 12 weeks gestation. Here is a very important piece of the advice: wear goggles because the fluid within the cysts are under pressure and love to get into residents' eyes! Our Thursdays are pretty busy because it is fibroid day. Grossing fibroids is not complicated - they are just difficult because fibroids can be hard to cut and you need multiple blades handy. They need to be serially sectioned adequately to be sure there is no malignancy present, but it can be tedious at times.

I was on this rotation on Christmas Eve and of course received a pelvic exenteration on top of the normal grossing load. This is a radical surgical procedure that removes a person's bladder, urethra, rectum, anus, and possibly prostate or vagina, cervix, uterus, ovaries, vulva, and fallopian tubes. I was at the hospital grossing until 9 p.m. and was exhausted by the time I was done. Usually this wouldn't affect me but it was Christmas Eve and I wanted to go home. I missed midnight mass and a delicious family dinner. I didn't arrive until 11 p.m. but luckily everyone stayed up waiting for me and I was able to enjoy the last hour of Christmas Eve. Thank God, I was still close to home.

Hematology/ Hematopathology

This rotation covers bone marrows, peripheral bone smears, coagulation, complete blood count tests, and hemoglobinopathies. In the mornings, we go over the slides of the abnormal blood count tests. Many of these cases were abnormal due to lymphoma, leukemias, and infections. Oddly enough, we actually had a case of Babesia, a malaria-like disease from a person who visited Long Island. Once you see it on a slide it is hard to forget it. The early afternoons are spent signing out bone marrow biopsies. The late afternoons are spent signing out coagulation studies and hemoglobinopathies. In your board application, they will ask how many bone marrows were performed by you.

Cytogenetics

Cytogenetics is one of our clinical pathology rotations and its use is continuously growing as chromosomal abnormalities and identification of syndromes expand. It is an essential diagnostic and prognostic tool in various branches of medicine especially in oncology and pediatrics. Our program concentrates on cancer cytogenetics and we are responsible for gaining experience in identifying human chromosomes, becoming familiarized with cytogenetic techniques and nomenclature and how to interpret and report structural chromosome abnormalities. At the end of the rotation, we feel confident about being able to interpret genetic tests, karyotypes and fluorescent in situ hybridization (FISH) analyses.

Community Hospital

The residents are sent to a small community Hospital in New Jersey to gain exposure to community pathology. Community pathology makes up the majority of pathology jobs. This hospital has a private practice of 5 pathologists that lease space from the hospital and is responsible for both anatomic and clinical pathology. There is a clinic which houses pathologist, radiologists, surgeons, nurses, and social workers under one roof, so in a sense it is a one stop shopping for patient. Here the pathologist performs fine needle aspirations of breast, thyroid, and basically anything that can have a needle stuck through it. In this model, the pathologist sees the patient, does the aspiration, and within 10 minutes the specimen is stained and given a diagnosis. Once a week, the entire clinic meets and discusses malignant cases. The collegiate interaction between the pathologist, radiologists, and surgeons helps improve patient care as they elaborate on the care of a single patient. This rotation helped me to identify the importance of interacting with clinicians and discussing the care of the patient.

Forensic Pathology

I had this rotation during my third year at the New York City Medical Examiner's office. The autopsies done at the Medical Examiner's are completely different from the ones done at the hospital and I ended up loving the rotation. This rotation makes you appreciate everyday that goes by without anything happening to you. One of my cases was a 32-year-old female who suddenly died coming out of the subway which happened to be at my train station. She was on her way to work thinking nothing was wrong and then just suddenly died! It hits a little too close to home because that could be anyone including me! This rotation also makes you think twice without doing risky things. For example, one of our patient's was a 52-year-old male who is thought he could across the street in time. At the same time there was a truck who didn't see him rushing through and hit him causing multiple lower extremity fractures which led to exsanguination and his eventual death. I now just always just wait for the light to change instead of rushing in; it's just not worth it!

Exams

In order to sit for the anatomical/clinical pathology boards, you need to complete 18 months of anatomical pathology and 18 months of clinical pathology. Anatomic pathology includes Autopsy, Pediatric Pathology, Cytopathology, Dermatopathology, Forensic Pathology, Hematopathology, Neuropathology, Gastrointestinal Pathology and Gynecological Pathology while clinical pathology rotations include Chemical Pathology, Hematology, Blood Banking/Transfusion Medicine, Microbiology, Medical Microscopy, Informatics, Laboratory Management, and Molecular Pathology. For the anatomical component, most residents like using *Anatomic Pathology Board Review* by Jay H. Lefkowitch. I haven't started studying for my boards yet but this is the book I use during my anatomical rotations, and found the question in answer format easy to go through. For the clinical pathology towards, many residents use the *ASCP's Quick Compendium of Clinical Pathology*, which is in outline form. I personally think you also need to get a microbiology atlas for color pictures to do well on the boards.

Every year there is a Resident In-Service Examination (RISE) exam in the spring which can help assess where you are in your training and study for the board exams. Most programs don't have it count towards anything, but some programs use it as a formal evaluation and if that's the case you really need to prepare and study for the exam.

Personal Life

Being in pathology does lend to having a personal life more than other subspecialties, however, this is still medicine and we do have to give up the occasional weekend or weeknight. We don't have early morning rounds like most of the residents do; we just have a mandatory 8 a.m. didactic conference. If you are motivated, you can still have time to go to the gym in the morning or after work. The time I get to leave the hospital depends on the rotation I'm on. For example, a clinical rotation might be done by 5 pm while a surgical rotation can keep me at the hospital until 10 at night. Our hours at the hospital may not be as long as other specialties, but we have to spend longer amounts of time reading and preparing for conferences at home.

As far as vacation goes, I would love to say that I

visit exotic places but the truth is that 'stay-cations' are the norm. Living in New York is expensive and I still have all of my loans to pay up. Luckily, there is enough to do in the city and you learn which museums have free admission on a particular day.

Onward to Fellowship and the Job Market

Pathology is getting more competitive so subspecialization is probably warranted. For competitive specialties like dermatology, gastrointestinal, and forensic pathology you may need to start thinking about them in your first year. Applying for these fellowships starts about two years in advance. The fellowship process is still unorganized and plans on having a standardized fellowship application is still being debated. I applied for my oncologic pathology fellowship in October of my third year, received in invitation for an interview in February, and had my interview in early March. I actually only went on one interview and again it was a low stress, friendly process. I was offered the fellowship on the next day and gladly accepted! This is a one year fellowship that begins in July and then I will be looking for a job.

Pathology is a small specialty, so word of mouth and the reputation that you earn is very important in finding a job. According to the American Society for Clinical Pathology, 40% of the residents surveyed were pursuing a job in a community group practice. The average starting salary (excluding benefits) varies from $150,000 to $250,000 (43%); 36% were offered $100,000–$150,000; and 12% were offered less than $100,000. Even in today's unstable economy, all of the fellows at my program that were looking for a job have a position lined with up for next year. There are slight fluctuations from year to year but in general, the pathology job market continues to be strong.

References:

ASCP Pathology Resident Handbook 2008-2009.

ACGME Program Requirements for Graduate Medical Education in Anatomic Pathology and Clinical Pathology

CAREER SNAPSHOT

IN FOCUS: PATHOLOGY

Years in graduate school: 4 years medical school

Years in post-graduate training: 3-4 years residency

Fellowship: blood/banking/transfusion medicine, hematology, forensic pathology, etc.

Salary: average annual salary ranges from $240,000 to $330,000 and up

Pros: Expertise in every area of medicine, variable amount of patient interaction

Cons: May have limited patient interaction, possible heavy workload

Extra info: residency can be done in combined anatomic/clinical pathology program (4 years) or separate (3 years each)

Information taken from http://www.aamc.org/cim

"Veterinarians: Doctors Who Treat *More* Than Just One Species"

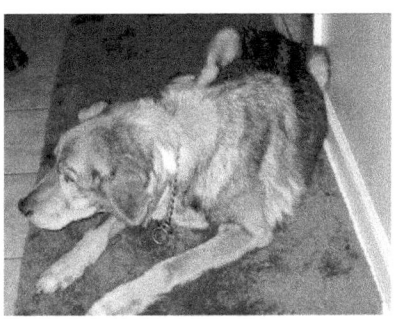

Joya S. Griffin, D.V.M.
Dermatology Resident
Cornell University Hospital for Animals

IN THIS CHAPTER...

* How fulfilling is it to work with animals?

* What steps are necessary in pursuing a veterinary degree?

* What standardized tests are needed for vet school?

* How is a medical residency different from veterinary residency?

* How demanding is a veterinarian's life?

Dr. Griffin, what first drew you to veterinary medicine? Why have you chosen to work with animals for a living?

Since I was a child I always had a connection with animals. I had many pets ranging from cats and dogs to turtles and frogs. I watched the movie Dr. Doolittle (the original) and fell in love with the idea of talking to the animals and curing all that ailed them. As I got older, I excelled in school and enjoyed math and science courses. It therefore seemed appropriate to combine my academic strengths and my love for four-footed creatures.

What was the most difficult part of the vet school admission/application process?

The hardest part of applying to veterinary school was the fact that I was a minority in a sea of pre-meds. No one knew the specific courses I needed to take, or what schools I should apply to. I felt like I was doing everything on my own. I had mentoring from a lab animal veterinarian at the Johns Hopkins Medical Institute, and there were a few books that served as a listing of individual school requirements. Otherwise, the whole thing was a learning process for me and my professors.

Tell us about your interview and testing experiences.

Vet schools require either the MCAT (Medical College Admissions Test) or GRE (Graduate Record Examination). I chose to take the GRE. The test takes about 3-4 hours, and they have questions examining verbal reasoning, quantitative reasoning, and analytical writing. I participated in

VETWARD Bound, a summer enrichment program for minority students interested in veterinary medicine. It was offered at Michigan State University the summer before my senior year in college, and during this 8-week long program, I took a GRE preparatory course that helped me to review material and practice simulated tests. At the end of the summer, I took the GRE and was fairly happy with my score.

As far as interviewing, Cornell Vet School is one of the few vet colleges that does not interview. They also accept their class by January of each year, so I had already been accepted to Cornell before I interviewed at any other school. I did interview at Ohio State University; this was a two-part interview, one with a professor and the other with the Dean of Admissions. Both interviews were fairly laid back and aimed at my personal attributes, goals, and what I was looking for in a vet school. I chose to attend Cornell and have been very happy with that decision.

What is the application process like for vet school/residency? Have you overcome any major obstacles in your pursuit of residency training?

Veterinary medicine differs from human medicine in that a graduate from vet school is not required to do an internship or residency in order to practice. Many recent graduates go directly into private practice. However, if a person wants to specialize in something other than general medicine, they must do a one-year internship in medicine and surgery before applying for a residency program. Most residency programs range from 2-3 years and some programs, like surgery and cardiology, require a specialty internship.

Most vet students who are interested in residency apply through the VRIMP (Veterinary Residency and Internship Matching Program). These programs mostly consist of equine internships, though some programs do not go through the match. I applied for an internship and matched at a large private practice in Chicago. After my year there I applied for a dermatology residency through the VIRMP and did not match. Fortunately, a position was created for me at my vet school (Cornell) which allowed me to return and train for my residency in veterinary dermatology.

What was the transition to residency like? How long did it take to settle into the position/routine?

The transition to residency was fairly painless since I was returning to Cornell. I was comfortable with the routine and the faculty I was working with. Internship in Chicago was more painful and required many, many thankless hours with little respect. That was a hard year, but residency itself has been lots of fun.

Give a detailed description of a day in your life.

Monday through Thursday, the residents receive cases with vet students. Most of these are small animal cases (dogs or cats). We round with the students over the cases they have seen on Tuesday and Thursday afternoons, and also Wednesday and Friday mornings. Wednesday and Friday mornings are also reserved for skin testing and any procedures such as farm calls, biopsy, or sedated ear flush. Monday mornings and Friday afternoons are set aside for resident training. During my first year, chapter review from three major texts was done on Monday mornings. On Friday afternoons of my second year, I spent time doing histopathology unknowns. Thursday afternoons we spend 2 hours at the multi-headed scope reviewing histopathology cases sent in from outside practitioners. A general day lasts from 8 or 9 in the morning until 5:30 or 6 p.m.

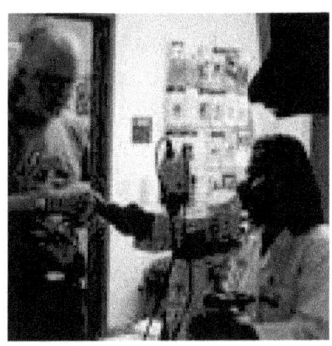

How have you managed the sickest patients you encountered? What helped you through those times?

Luckily, now that I am a resident I rarely have in-patients; as an intern, other overnight doctors and our criticalists helped manage our critical patients.

How do you manage your time? Your family? Friends? Relationships?

Time management is very difficult, mostly because I feel like I have been in school my entire life. I went from high school, to college, to vet school, and now I'm still working hard in residency. I'm glad that my schedule is predominantly 9-5 now, so I try to enjoy my life a lot more and make up for lost time. I do have a long-distance relationship which keeps me busy and out of town often. Although I find myself being easily distracted, I try to get as much done during the week because weekends are often filled with my much-needed extra-curricular activities.

Are you active in any advocacy organizations? State health organizations? What role does community service play in your career?

I was Co-president of VOICE my second year in vet school, and as Co-President I was responsible for the new name of the group. VOICE stands for *Vet students as One In Culture and Ethnicity* and is a group that focuses on celebrating and educating the veterinary community on cultural and ethnic diversity.

The group was started, under a different name, two years prior by a couple of vet students. My class, which had a larger group of minorities in it (5 African American women, 3 African American males, 3 Asians, and 4 Latinas) was very excited about this group and strived to make it more visible in the vet school community. I changed its name in order to make it a group that was easy to remember and that "spoke" for the people. During our year in charge, we hosted movie nights, a mentorship program with pre-vet students at Cornell undergrad, and organized several taste fairs (one for black history month, Latino month, and Asian History month). We also had a Latin Dance Night that was very well attended.

The group has continued to be successful and went national 2 years ago. There are several chapters at vet schools around the country, and the charter chapters have received start-up funds from Pfizer Animal Health. So for me and my executive board, VOICE was our baby. We loved it and what it represented. It gave students of culture a place and forum to be comfortable in and to voice their concerns. Many students who are not considered minorities are also active members.

VOICE National Website.....lots of historical info on here as well as list of current chapters. http://www.vetvoice.org/index-2.html

Did you spend any time abroad or do any rotating clerkships? Why?

Yes. As a vet student I spent several weeks externing at different practices, private and academic. I did this because I wanted to look at different internship and residency possibilities.

Name some things that have surprised or disappointed you about residency.

Because I was able to come back to Cornell for residency, I thought things would be like they were when I was here as a student. However, being in the role as a resident, you don't have time to socialize and have fun like you did as a student. My program only has two residents, but I don't even spend time with my fellow resident, or the ones in other programs. Because my program doesn't have in-patients, I don't interact with the residents that spend time working in the hospital after hours and on weekends. I've found that each vet program is very isolated amongst itself. Life in general as a vet resident has been very isolated.

What has been your most valuable resource in this process? What administrators have helped you along?

Cornell has been a very loving and supportive environment for me; they really want each student to succeed. The school is decentralized so that everything you need as a student is within the vet college itself. This is important, because it makes you more than just a face down in the financial aid office. The faculty and staff really know each student and that helped a lot when going through the academic years. The faculty is easily accessible and approachable.

Are you happy with your post-graduate choices? What other areas/fields have you ever looked into?

I am very happy with my career choice. I love dermatology and am excited to practice what I like and at the same time have a life.

Tell us about death, marriage, birth, or major life-changing experiences you have had.

My mother died of cancer in between my second and third year of vet school. The vet college - including faculty, staff and students - was so supportive. I was able to take time off at the beginning of the semester to be with my family, and make up the course work and exams before the semester ended. The love and support I had honestly made it possible for me to even come back to school after that experience.

How was your education financed? What are your plans to repay your debt, if necessary?

Federal loans, unfortunately. I am going to pay off my debt as slowly as possible. It is daunting at times; luckily I have not had to pay it back during my internship and residency years....but repayment is soon impending.

What outside interests are you pursuing?

My biggest current goal is to pass my boards in August so that I can be a board-certified veterinary dermatologist. No time for any outside interests for now. I do one day hope to be married, and one day further into the future, the mother of three and a possible ☺

What are your future aspirations? What do you want your practice to look like in 10 years? Have you started to look into job positions?

Next year I will be co-chief of the dermatology service at Cornell, which consists of training students for 6 months out of the year in the clinics and lecturing to them during their dermatology course. After this one-year stint, I plan on going into private practice. I do enjoy academia; however, do not want to live in Ithaca my entire life, so I'll be looking to do this elsewhere.

CAREER SNAPSHOT

IN FOCUS: VETERINARY MEDICINE

Years in graduate school: 4 years veterinary school

Years in post-graduate training: 1-2 years residency optional

Residency: avian medicine, equine medicine and surgery, zoological medicine, etc.

Salary: average annual salary ranges from $60,000 to $90,000 and up

Pros: work with animals in a variety of settings

Cons: lower average salary than medicine or dentistry

Extra info: employment in this field is expected to increase 35% through 2016

Information taken from http://www.collegegrad.com

"You Don't Have To Brush Your Teeth - Just The Ones You Want To Keep"

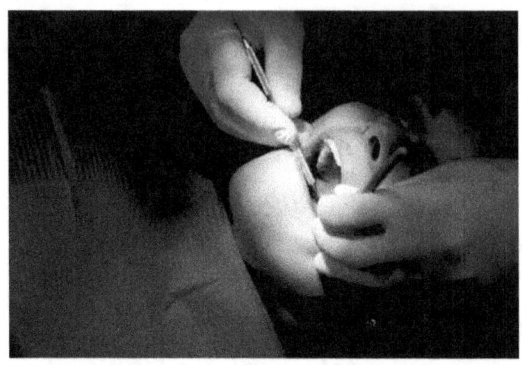

Elo C. Adibe, D.M.D.
Staff Prosthodontist
Veterans Affairs Medical Center,
Philadelphia, PA

IN THIS CHAPTER...

- How is dental school set up?

- What residencies and fellowships are possible after completing dental school?

- What is the life of a dentist like?

- How can a dentist get involved in community work?

Why did you go into dentistry Dr. Adibe? What appealed to you about the field?

I liked the idea of having a job that would put me in a position to help people. I have always liked working with my hands, and I also liked the fact that I would have time to spend with my family. In fact, I would have more control over my time in general.

Your father, brother, and sister are all in the health professions - did you feel that you had to go into something similar? Did you feel pressure to go into a science-related field?

No. I actually didn't feel any pressure at all. My father is a physician, I knew that my brother wanted to be a physician, but when I finished college, my sister wasn't sure of what she wanted to go into. I was looking for something to do, but there really wasn't anything that I was passionate about at the time. I didn't like anything else and couldn't see myself going down other career paths. I didn't even start off with a passion for dentistry – that didn't come until after my second or third year of dental school. It started off as something I wanted to check out. I liked it, but I didn't love it. After spending some time in the field, now I truly love the actual work. I love doing lab work, prosthetics, planning cases – the whole thing. My particular job enables me to focus on the artistic side of dentistry and really make a difference in someone's life. I think I would do it for free – if only those bills didn't keep coming!

How does dental school work? What classes do you take?
What rotations do you do?

For the first two years of dental school, we do
mainly didactic work – a lot like medical school.
We take classes like microbiology, physiology,
biochemistry, microanatomy, histology, gross
anatomy – a lot of the same courses as medical
school. We just don't take genetics. There is a
strong focus on head and neck information, but we
do learn about the upper extremities, upper body,
heart, and lungs, etc. In addition to classes we have
our pre-clinic, where we basically work on
mannequins. We work on developing our lab skills.
We take a lot of tests, and then for the last two years
of school, we are in rotations – again, a lot like
medical school.

How did you decide on the school you attended?

I didn't apply to many dental schools – mostly places around the Northeast. I applied to Howard, Maryland, New Jersey Dental School, Temple, and maybe some others. I got into a couple of these schools, but NJDS was the cheapest since I was considered an in-state student. Also I knew some people who were attending that institution for medical school - like my brother and other friends – and that made it much easier to make the decision.

How was your education financed?

My father paid for it. I was one of the lucky ones.

Other than pre-clinic and classes, what kinds of things did you do in dental school?

I did a lot of volunteer work in school, mainly through student organizations like the Student National Dental Association. I did it around the communities of East Orange and Newark in New Jersey – places around my school. I definitely had a passion for it, but I also got involved in order to make my resume more impressive. I was in student government, a class representative for a course or two, and I tutored in some classes. Also, some of our classes required that we go to area elementary schools to do demonstrations on proper oral care.

How was your social life during school?

I didn't have much of one. I was with my girlfriend, now wife, the whole time that I was in dental school, and I was working so hard that I barely had time to really party.

What about time management? How did you deal with that?

It is very important to manage your time. It's key. The better you are at that, the more successful you'll be in any type of academic environment. You'll be more efficient with studying and everything else. I wasn't that great with time management, so I probably had a harder time in school than other people probably did. Those who were more disciplined and organized than I was were able to focus on the important stuff instead of always playing catch-up. Maybe if I did that better I would've had more of a social life. I always tell people that dental school was the worst 4 years of my life, probably because of poorly managed time and resources. Luckily I made it through that – albeit the hard way - but now, I love dentistry.

What standardized tests are taken in dental school?

We have the Dental Aptitude Test, or DAT, in order to get into dental school. After your second year, you take Step 1 of the national board exams. Then sometime during fourth year you take Step 2. Step 1 is the more important test because that's the one that a lot of post graduate programs look at to determine acceptance. I studied on my own for those tests, and I used all of the study materials available for purchase out there. I did alright on Step 1; Step 2 – eh, I passed. I actually liked those standardized tests because they put everyone on equal playing ground. There were some people that seemed to be on top of their game according to class ranks, but when they take the exams, they didn't do as well as expected. I believe that if you did what you were supposed to do in class during the first two years, it'll show up on those standardized tests. It's a great way to validate your position and know that you're learning what you need for graduation.

Have you been surprised by anything during your journey through dentistry?

I can't say that I've been too surprised. It definitely wasn't easy – it was very difficult. I went into it thinking it was going to be hard, but I really didn't know what to expect. I took it as it came and dealt with it all.

I did learn that there are a lot of things you have to contend with. It was a surprise how subjective parts of dental school can be. For instance, when you take a gross anatomy or biochemistry test, the answers are what they are. You take the test, you get graded, and that's that. However in the pre-clinic or regular clinic, you have a professor that's judging your work and deciding your entire grade. One professor may say one thing and another professor may say another thing. You can do something exactly the same way as another student, but the same professor may give two people two different grades for something similar. That was a surprise to me, and it can create major problems.

Although they are trying to take steps to correct that problem, I wouldn't even know what to do about something like that. It's unfortunate to say it, but a lot of times, I think about being a black man in those situations. You do your work, but since it's graded subjectively, you may want to pull the race card when you don't understand why a certain grade was given. In that type of environment, and given the history of dentistry (we had to form the National Dental Association because we were not allowed into the American Dental Association), thoughts of old timers being responsible for our grades can mess with you. Am I being graded harshly because I'm black, or is my work really sub par? Why did the student next to me get a significantly better grade than I did when we worked together and submitted the same work? That can eat you up inside, and I would say that was a true shock when I got into dentistry.

What happens after dental school? General practice? Residency? Fellowship?

When I graduated, there was the option to go out and work in private practice, or to do some sort of residency. Most people opt to do some sort of a residency; there may be a select few that go right into private practice. As far as residencies are concerned, there's the general practice residency which is usually a year, sometimes it can be two years. In addition to that, there are a good number of dental specialties. Periodontics - basically gum surgery – is usually 3 years, Oral Maxillofacial Surgery is the long one – it's a four to six year residency where you have the option of getting your M.D. as well. Endodontics is the root canal specialty, and it is 2-3 years, Prosthodontics, which is what I do, takes 3 years, Orthodontics takes care of braces and is 2-3 years. In addition to these, there is public health dentistry, oral medicine, oral radiology, pediatric dentistry (which is gaining a lot of popularity), and oral pathology.

We do have some fellowships, but I don't know a lot of them, because once you do your specialty, it's rare to go onto fellowship. The ones that I'm familiar with are in my specialty. There's oral maxillofacial prosthetics which deals with the mouth, nose, ears, and sometimes fixing the palate. They also do repositioning devices for people undergoing radiation treatments for head and neck cancer.

What exactly do you do each day? Are you involved in cleanings, fillings, root canals, or other things?

A prosthodontist is the dental specialist that deals with the replacement of missing teeth. We do this either through crown and bridge work, dentures, or implants to support and retain prostheses. I work at the VA hospital, and most of the time I'm working on implants, crowns and bridges, and dentures. As far as fillings, if I think that my case will move along quicker by doing one, instead of pausing work to send a patient to a general dentist, then I'll do it myself. Same thing with root canals – every now and then, if I think it's going to help out the larger treatment plan for a particular patient, I'll do that too. Cleanings aren't a part of my specialty, so I haven't done one in years.

What is your work week like?

Right now I work Monday through Thursday at the hospital. I used to work Fridays and Saturdays at a private office, but those work hours vary. Sometimes I would work every other week, other times it could be once a month. It all depends on how business is. I work pretty hard, but I don't feel like my job is taking away from time with my family.

Do you work with any students in your job now? What is it like to work with them?

Yes. I spend some time as an attending at the VA hospital, and I work with the general practice residents when they're doing something involving implants. I enjoy it a lot. It makes me realize how much information I have in my head. It reinforces certain things that I already know. Also there's the gratification of helping somebody out, of helping students and residents get through a difficult time. I hope to stay involved in teaching in one form or another regardless of where dentistry takes me in the future.

What do you want your life to look like in 10 years?

I'd like to be at the VA – not full time, maybe a day or two per week. I want to have at least two practices where I split my time. I want to teach and give lectures. I'd like to be a clinical professor working closely with students. I'll do continuing education (CE) courses, ensuring that I'll always get better at my job. I want to try to be the best prosthodontist that I can be.

Do you have any advice for students entering dental school now or thinking about dentistry?

Don't piss anyone off because a lot of dentistry is subjective! Unfortunately you have to play it like it's a game. Study hard. Work the game. Do what you have to do in order to get out. Make sure that whatever you do is legal! There is a lot of cheating that goes on in dental school. As with anything though, some people get caught and get a slap on the wrist. Others get caught and sit through round table meetings where administrators try to find the quickest way to kick them out. You don't want to be in that situation, so work hard and do what is asked of you.

CAREER SNAPSHOT

IN FOCUS: DENTISTRY

Years in graduate school: 4 years dental school

Years in post-graduate training: 1-6 years residency optional

Residency: endodontics, orthodontics, prosthodontics, oral radiology, etc.

Salary: average annual salary ranges from $150,000 to $190,000 and up

Pros: once established, may work 35-40 hours per week

Cons: expensive dental supplies and equipment

Extra info: a dentist can also obtain a M.D. degree through a combined oral maxillofacial residency program

Information taken from http://www.collegegrad.com

"Life Is Good…*Now*"

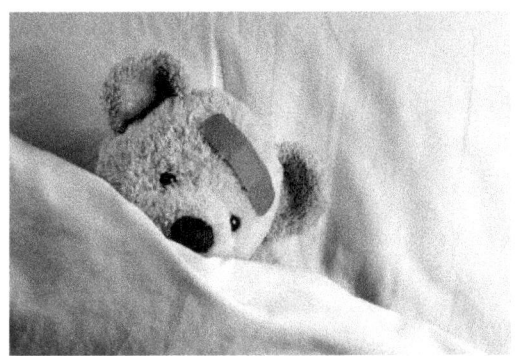

Adonia H. Dibbell, M.D.
PGY-3, Lewis M. Fraad Department of Pediatrics
Jacobi Medical Center/Albert Einstein College
of Medicine, Bronx, NY

IN THIS CHAPTER...

* What is the life of a pediatrician like?

* What is it like to work with children?

* How can one deal with family, friends, relationships, *and* medicine?

* What sacrifices are needed to succeed in medicine?

Dr. Dibbell, what kind of doctor are you? What does your job entail?

I am a pediatrician. Pediatricians work with newborn babies up to the age of 21 in some cases. In residency we learn about dealing with the medical illnesses of children and adolescents, as well as dealing with the social aspects of medicine. We learn to be sensitive to the unique experience children and their families have in the hospital.

What's the best part of your job? The worst part?

The kids are definitely the best part. They are fun and they make me smile all the time. It makes the day go by quicker. I feel like I'm helping them start their life right and helping their families get through an anxious and difficult period in their child's life. Perhaps I'm not making the biggest difference in their life overall, but I'm definitely helping in that moment. As far as the worst part of residency in my opinion, it's the hours! I like my sleep, so when I don't get enough, that's hard to deal with.

Why did you go into medicine? When did you make the decision to really pursue this as a career?

I have always liked science and was good at it. I don't think I could have seen myself doing anything that wasn't science related - then again, I only knew about doctors and lawyers while growing up. In college, I explored some ideas about other fields, but I crossed them out one by one in my head. I didn't actually try other things in depth in school, but luckily, I ended up with something great.

How did you go about your pursuit of medicine? What decisions did you make to set you up for a spot? How did you know what to do?

I always knew I wanted to be a doctor and was always focused on getting good grades. I received scholarships to college, and continued studying really hard. The school I ended up at was really focused on medicine, and their pre-med program was excellent. They guided students through the application process and had valuable resources available. Because of that, I did well on the MCAT (Medical College Admissions Test) and got my application in on time.

What was your thought process in choosing a medical school? How did you choose your residency program? What about the job search?

I actually regret going to the medical school I went to. I chose a school with an impressive name, thinking it would be better in terms of getting me into residency or being a better doctor. I should have gone to the school that gave me the most money. In reality, it's all about your loans in the end – the name of a school doesn't guarantee a great education or good experience.

As far as residency, I always liked working with kids. The only other specialty I was interested in was anesthesia, but I tried it and it wasn't a good fit for me. I did a two week rotation and found myself not liking it as much as my pediatric rotations. Then I did even more peds rotations, and pretty soon, the decision was clear to me.

My residency program definitely was not my top choice, but I liked the fact that everyone was so supportive of one another. The attendings were very personable and you could talk to them about anything. Coming from my medical school, which was very academic, it was nice to be in a more relaxed atmosphere.

For the job search after residency, I just went on different websites. The bad thing about my program is that they don't have a big network, so I had to go onto the AAP (American Academy of Pediatrics) website and get interviews from there. Other residents in my program sent out emails about jobs available, and that was very effective.

What did you give up for medicine?

In medical school, you're about 22-26 years old, and that's the time in your life when you're allowed to be young and free. In college, I worked so hard that I didn't have the stereotypical experience where I partied, made mistakes, and took chances. Then I got to med school and wanted to go out more. It's hard though, because we have to be so focused on becoming a doctor. You see your friends – other young people your age – who are doing other things, and who have all their weekends off. They don't have to study, and they are making more than a decent living.

I knew that my time in medical school and residency was temporary, but my youth was not. I gave up that experience that most young college graduates have post-college. But now I realize I am going to have so much time to have many more wonderful experiences in the future, and I only see that now that my time in residency is ending.

What did you gain along the way?

Thanks to medicine, I have a good career that I'll enjoy for the rest of my life and will be able to financially support myself and my family. I've realized that you have to really like medicine in order to be successful in it. It's hard and it's painful at times, but I'm happy with my job now and have come to terms with the sacrifices made.

Any surprises along the way? How did you get over them?

I was surprised by how much I hated my first year of residency. I really, really wanted to quit. I was tired all the time. I didn't feel like I was learning; I felt more like a secretary. I didn't have a life – I would just go to work and go home. I was cranky and mean. I didn't want to speak to anybody. It affected my relationships, and it was a very painful time. If it wasn't for my mother I wouldn't have made it through. Also, knowing that I had so many loans and needed a good job to pay them off, I figured I just had to put up with the long hours. I'm glad I didn't quit because it has gotten easier over the years, and now I'm almost done.

What is most important to you in keeping your sanity?

Right now, things are fine. I'm a third year resident with fewer hours to put in. It is not as hard, and now I feel like I know more stuff. It's definitely not easy but I feel like things are better since intern year is over. I am happy now, and that's most important to my sanity.

How do you deal with family, friends, and everything in your life in addition to medicine?

In going into medicine you have to be so focused on it that you can't deal with everyone else's drama. I had to 'x' some people out of my life for a time because I personally couldn't deal with everything. I was really only concerned with my immediate family and everyone else's problem was not my problem. My mother was very supportive during that time. She would do whatever, whenever I needed it. She would cook for me, clean for me, and take me places. My brother was also very supportive. I had two people that were there for me no matter what, and I didn't have the rest of my family bothering me.

The good thing about my friends is that most of them were in med school and residency with me, so they were going through the same things. We would hang out while studying, and get through tests and difficult classes together. Medicine did affect my relationship with an ex-boyfriend though. Because I was so upset and cranky, I would get mad over very little things. I don't think I realized how much it affected my personality at the time.

What do you want to do with your medical degree?

I'm not too sure yet. I have a job lined up for after residency, but it's shift work and I don't think I could do a job like that for the rest of my life. I'm not sure if I want to do a fellowship or if I'll be happy with a private practice job in the future. I like seeing patients and building good relationships. I like problem solving, but I kind of want something more interesting than primary care. At this point, I feel like I need time to not work so hard for once in my life. To not be studying all the time. To not work 80 hours a week. After that, I'll see what I actually want to do.

Any last minute advice for aspiring doctors?

It is a very, very difficult journey to go through. Looking back, I don't know if I would do it again – knowing what I know now with all the loans and fees and time and sacrifice. I can say that I am happy with my job now, and with what I have accomplished. I am very proud of what I've done, and I think in the end you'll be happy with what you're doing if you go into medicine. My advice is to talk to people in the field in order to understand what you're going to give up. If you look at all options and consider your choices carefully, you can have a great career in medicine, just like I do.

CAREER SNAPSHOT

IN FOCUS: PEDIATRICS

Years in graduate school: 4 years medical school

Years in post-graduate training: 3 years residency

Fellowship: adolescent medicine, neonatal medicine, pediatric emergency medicine, etc.

Salary: average annual salary ranges from $140,000 to $200,000 and up

Pros: shorter residency required, can make a difference early in children's lives

Cons: lower salary range, deal with frantic parents

Extra info: average number of hours worked per week is 49.4

Information taken from http://www.aamc.org/cim

"Is It A Rash?"

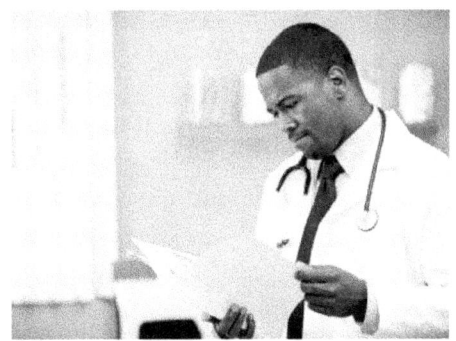

Richard H. Huggins, M.D.
PGY-2, Department of Dermatology
Henry Ford Hospital, Detroit, MI

IN THIS CHAPTER...

* What is the field of dermatology like?

* How hard is it to get into a dermatology residency?

* What are the options if one does not match into a specialty?

* How important is mentoring? How can one fit community service in with medicine?

* Does one have any fun while pursuing medicine?

Why did you go into medicine?

I went into medicine because I always liked biology and helping people. Actually, before I thought of medicine, I initially wanted to do research. There you can devote yourself to biology and do something beneficial for large populations. The only problem is that you don't get the same personal interaction as you do in medicine. You don't get to see the people that you're helping everyday and see exactly how they're benefiting from what you're doing. So with that in mind, it kind of steered me in the direction of medicine. Plus, the career path for medicine was more structured than research, and you get paid a lot more!

What kind of student were you in college and medical school, and what kind of resident are you now?

The thing that has helped me most in school and in my career is the fact that I can find interest in just about anything. Also, I have a very good memory. When I was in high school, if I just paid attention to everything in the classroom and asked questions, I never really had to study in order to do well. I didn't develop the best study habits back then because I didn't have to.

I carried the same poor study habits to college, but being bombarded with the rigorous workload at Johns Hopkins, that wasn't enough. I had to start refining my study skills and habits. It took me a little while, but by the end of my time in college I was used to putting in 10-12 hour study days on consecutive days when I needed to. I knew what I needed to do so that I could learn and retain a large amount of information. I ended up doing very well in the end of college, and then in medical school I decided ahead of time that I wanted to take things to an even higher level.

I didn't want to start off as slowly as I did in college because my mediocre grades in the beginning didn't give me the best G.P.A. I didn't want that to be the case in medical school, and I even took two years off after graduating. During that time I developed a more mature approach to my education, and was a lot more focused early on in med school. There is a lot more information you need to learn in medical school, and you have to do it a lot faster, all while the teachers teach you a lot less. So it's not that I came into med school right away and was able to do well off the bat, but I was motivated early on and I put the necessary time in. I refined my study skills and became extraordinarily efficient. I pursued other interests and again, was able to do well.

During my internship – the year of general medicine between finishing medical school and beginning derm residency - I did much more reading and work in dermatology than internal medicine because I knew that medicine was not where my career was going to end up. Then, in doing a dermatology research fellowship for two years after internship, my reading was directed towards preparing papers and completing research. Because of that, I haven't yet developed my residency study habits. I know that I'll find it a lot easier to absorb the information in derm, since it's all going to be directed at learning about the field that I want to be involved in for the rest of my life.

It'll help me to take better care of my patients and whatever I learn at night is going to directly apply to what I'll be doing during every day.

What career options did you think about – other than medicine and other than dermatology?

From the time that I was in the fifth grade and heard about genes and DNA, I wanted to do genetics research. From that time until my junior year in college, that's what I thought I was meant to do with my life. However, after exploring the field a little more and seeing the reality of doing research, it seemed that medicine fit me a lot more.

I decided on dermatology much later on. When I first started thinking about medicine, I wanted to do obstetrics and gynecology, just because I feel that I am able to connect with women. There are many women in my family and female friends who have benefited from their relationships with their doctors, and I thought that I could be a part of that. As I went through medical school and actually started thinking about the reality of doing something like OB-GYN, I realized that it just wouldn't be the best fit for me, given what I want to do with the rest of my life outside of medicine. My impression of the field was that you have to be in the hospital 80 hrs a week even after you're established in your career. Its stressful, you can get called in at any time, and I want to have a family that I'm around for. Also, I wanted to be involved in research and community service on some level. My options were limited by the fact that I only wanted to be in the hospital for a set amount of hours, so I kept searching.

The next field that I thought about was radiology. Here you have a good lifestyle and you get paid well, but I'm much more of a people person. That's what brought me to medicine in the first place, so obviously, the limited patient interaction of radiology wouldn't be for me either.

Dermatology floated through my mind a few times, but I always thought that it was only about acne and psoriasis. You give patients a few creams and send them on their way – nothing that I felt would be rewarding to me or make a big difference in someone's life. My mind wasn't changed until my pediatrics rotation, when we took care of a young girl who had a strange rash all over her body, from head to toe. No one in Peds knew what it was or how to treat it. We had to call in a dermatology consult, and their team came in, figured out that the rash was from an administered antibiotic, and advised us to find a more suitable medication. The rash quickly got better, and at the same time, the same girl who was very embarrassed about her appearance with the rash now came out of her shell. She didn't seem to care that she could have had a potentially dangerous medical condition, she just didn't want people to see her or come out of her room. Once the rash was gone, she felt more comfortable with others and even felt a lot better about herself. From that situation, I saw that dermatology was more than just acne. It reminded me of how important a person's appearance is to how they feel about themselves and how they relate to others. I saw that derm could be a challenge, it was a valuable profession, and I could feel good about working on skin cancer, vitiligo, and other perplexing conditions.

After exploring dermatology more, doing some research in the field, working in clinics, and seeing the day-to-day schedule, I appreciated that 1) there is a lot more to dermatology than simple rashes and acne, and 2) even the acne that a teenager may have may not be difficult to treat, but it may have a big effect on their quality of life. I knew this was something that would allow me to continue doing research and I wouldn't have to be in the hospital so many hours. I could spend time with my family and pursue lots of outside interests…So that was the beginning of my path to dermatology.

What did you do to ensure a residency spot in dermatology?

It took me three years to get my position in dermatology. Derm is probably the most competitive specialty in medicine - for a lot of the reasons that I was interested in it. The hours aren't that bad, there is a good lifestyle, a high salary, and you get to talk to patients everyday. So, the cream of the crop in most med school classes wants to do dermatology. I wasn't able to get accepted the first time that I applied and it took a lot of introspection and reflection to see what I could do to improve myself as an applicant and secure a position. This is what I wanted to do with my life and what I was passionate about, so I wanted to do whatever was necessary. I spoke to some of the program directors and department chairs that had interviewed me and not accepted me, just to get a feel for what I could do to better myself. One common theme that kept coming back was research, so that's what I did on the side during my internship. I did research and tried to get some more publications out there. When I didn't get accepted again after applying the second time, I decided to pursue a fellowship in clinical dermatology research, where I did derm research full time. My goal was to get those publications out there, get more experience in research, increase networking, and make more connections in dermatology. This would ultimately show programs that I was passionate about dermatology and willing to do whatever it took to get a position. Midway through my first year of research, I did finally get accepted into a residency program.

Tell us about the importance of mentoring, especially as a black man in the black community.

I grew up in a lower socioeconomic area – especially where I went to high school. A lot of the people I was in school with and the people I saw on the corners are still in the same places they were when I left. They weren't able to take advantage of the opportunities that were available, and never tried to do anything big in their lives. Thinking about the reason for that, I don't feel that I was so special that I overcame all of this by myself and they weren't able to – I think the reason I did well is because of the role models that I had within my family. There were so many people that exemplified the fact that if you valued education and worked hard in school, you could be successful.

I had examples of this in my life, and a lot of other people don't have that. A lot of the major role models we have out there as black males are the athletes, rappers, and singers you see on television – people in entertainment. Now it's great to find success in that way, but only so many people can be successful in those fields, and that's a well known fact. However, if you work hard in school and in life, you're pretty much guaranteed to be successful – it's not really a gamble. I feel like I had those role models in life that told me the truth about the world and showed me how to get the things I wanted in life. I just want to be that kind of example for others so that it's easier for them to see themselves being successful. If they take their education seriously and set realistic goals, they can do anything they want in life.

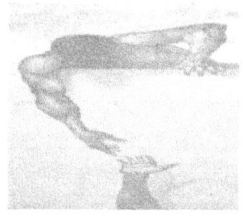

From the beginning of your schooling to the point you are now, did you have any fun along the way?

I had a lot of fun. My first year in college – even though I could have done better academically - was the most fun that I've ever had. A lot of that came from finally being around people who were intelligent and focused on what they wanted to do with their lives – not just taking classes because they were being forced to.

I think I had even more fun in medical school because I really had a lot in common with my classmates – we were all in medicine and could share every experience. We were all so much more motivated because you have to be in order to get through college and make it into medical school. I got lucky and met people who became good, good friends. We supported each other in our studies, got to complain to each other about things we didn't like, and even got involved in a lot of extra-curricular activities together. I was involved in the Student National Medical Association (SNMA) and took on a leadership role in helping and supporting other minority medical students and the larger community. This was the first time I took such an active leadership role, but it made med school that much more fun and exciting.

I found another important passion during this time, and that was mentoring. To realize that it was something I was very passionate about, and to be able to mentor others as a medical student - it made my med school career that much more fulfilling.

One of my biggest regrets from college was not being able to study abroad, so I came into medical school determined to make up for that. In the course of trying to learn about dermatology, I was able to go to Holland – a trip that was mostly paid for to study dermatology. My trip to Ethiopia was to study dermatology even more and get hands-on experience.

All in all, I would say that I had much more diverse experiences in medical school than I did in college, and it all amounted to lots of good times.

What do you ultimately want to do?

I haven't decided 100%. There are a lot of things I could do. One thing is ensure the financial security of the generations that come after me in my family. When I have children, I want to be able to provide for them and get them as many opportunities as I can. I'd like to have some money set aside so that when they get older it'll be easier for them to maneuver through life. I want to leave an imprint on my family for generations to come, and I even want to support my relatives in need now through college and private school.

Within dermatology, I'll work with the residency program and provide guidance to the medical students that come through the program. I want to be involved in research in my career, and be involved in the community. I've wanted to work in a free dermatology clinic, where people who don't have insurance and can't afford to get derm treatments are able to get what they need. Doing all of these things at the same time is going to be difficult, and I realize that I have to decide on what is most important. I'm going to have to prioritize what I want to focus on the most and what I'm not going to be able to pay as much attention to. I want to continue mentoring outside of dermatology – speaking to high school, elementary and college students in disadvantaged areas. Letting them know that they can do whatever they want to do is important to me, and trying to be there to support them through whatever is my goal.

Trying to do all of this is going to be tricky and I'm still trying to figure how to best balance it all out.

What's the one thing you wish that someone told you before starting on your journey?

Maybe that being smart isn't everything. To accomplish great things, being intelligent is definitely a good starting point, but that's not all there is to life. You have to have drive, you have to work hard, and you have to put your energy in the right direction. I wish I knew the importance of networking, knowing the right people, and finding the right people to speak to for advice. I think that if I had learned that earlier in my career, then it might have made things easier.

Do you have any last minute advice for students who are trying to get to where you are?

My best advice would be to seek out role models. Seek out people who have been through what you're trying to go through. If there are a lot of steps you have to take to get to where you want to go, ask someone who is there so that you know what the steps are. Try to be in touch constantly & faithfully with someone at each level - for example if you want to become a dermatologist, you need to talk with some dermatologists, derm residents, some medical students. Talk to people at the beginning and end of their careers, so you can benefit from people's experiences – both their mistakes and the things that went well for them. In the process of seeking out role models and finding out what people did before you - what worked for them and what didn't – don't feel that you have to do things exactly the same way. You can do something else. Take what advice you can, figure out what works for you, and what makes sense for you. Realize that there are a million different ways to reach the same end result. Don't be discouraged if you fall short along the way, because at every stage in my career I've made mistakes. Mistakes, failure, and success go hand in hand, because it's only a matter of a time before you fail. You'll probably fail a number of times, but it's all about what you do about it, how you learn from your mistakes, and how you persevere. Follow that advice and you'll have a good start to securing whatever career you want.

CAREER SNAPSHOT

IN FOCUS: DERMATOLOGY

Years in graduate school: 4 years medical school

Years in post-graduate training: 4 years residency

Fellowship: dermatopathology, pediatric dermatology

Salary: average annual salary ranges from $280,000 to $400,000 and up

Pros: overnight/in-house call often not required

Cons: stereotype that all your work relates to pimples and acne

Extra info: dermatologists often treat a number of sexually transmitted diseases

Information taken from http://www.aamc.org/cim

"You May Encounter Many Defeats, But You Must Not Be Defeated"
–Maya Angelou

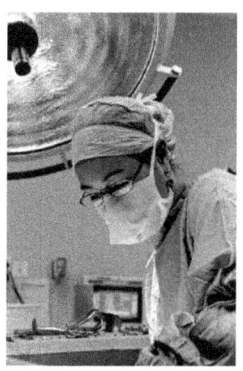

L. Efua Essandoh, M.D.
PGY-3, Department of Obstetrics and Gynecology
Bridgeport Hospital (affiliate of Yale
University), Bridgeport, CT

IN THIS CHAPTER...

* What are standardized tests in medicine like?

* What extracurricular opportunities are available in
medical school?

* What is an OB-GYN doctor? What does he/she do?

* How can one deal with a rigorous schedule?
Shortcomings during residency?

The Pursuit of Medicine: Is this really for me?

Dr. Essandoh, what first led you to pursue a career in medicine?

Hmmm – that's a hard question, because I don't really know. As a child I remember seeing "Save The Kids" commercials on television. I would constantly wonder about their sad faces and starving bodies, and wish for something meaningful that I could do for them. From that I initially thought I would end up working with kids in order to improve their situation. Later in life I became interested in pursuing social work, but since I liked science so much, I decided to combine all of my passions and give medicine a try. There was no one moment when I knew that medicine, or even obstetrics and gynecology, would be my choice, but looking back, it's crazy to me that I found something that so perfectly satisfies and challenges me everyday.

In medical school, what, other than class work, kept you busy?

I went to New Jersey Medical School (NJMS, part of the University of Medicine and Dentistry of New Jersey, UMDNJ), and did many things. I was on the Student Affairs Committee and worked with the American Medical Women's Association (AMWA). Above all, I love the Student National Medical Association (SNMA), and did a lot of work with that organization. SNMA is the nation's oldest and largest independent, student-run organization focused on the needs and concerns of medical students of color. Most medical schools across the country have a chapter, and we do so much to give back to the communities we come from. At NJMS we participated in lots of health fairs, and educated our student population about the importance of bone marrow donation and the dangers of lead poison. We did many projects with local undergraduate students – we talked to them about pursuing careers in the health sciences, and gave them the tips and tools to get them started with it.

I really loved our Big Sibling/Little Sibling (BigSib) program. This is where we pair second or third year medical students with an incoming first year. The upperclassman donates books and study material to their LittleSib, and stays with them throughout the year to ensure that they are excelling academically and socially. While giving school tours one day, I met a family that was concerned about their daughter who had been accepted to NJMS. They wanted to be sure that she would be happy at the school and be well prepared for residency. I made a promise that day to them that if she came to our school, I would take her under my wing as my LittleSib, and look out for her while she was a student. I promised that she would not only finish medical school, but she would match into the residency program of her choice and have a great time doing it. Once she matriculated, I passed on all of my classroom materials, and warned her about making the same mistakes I made. We formed a great bond, and to this day, we still talk often about medicine and about life. I traveled back to the school for her Match Day ceremony, and called her the night before she started residency. She is doing very well now, and I'm thrilled that I was able to be a guiding force in her academic career and play a small part in helping her achieve success.

Another thing that made me very happy while working with SNMA was our display case project. The organization had been assigned 3 or 4 large glass enclosures, with which we could display anything of our choosing. We presented information on different medical issues and the disparities seen in our present health care system, but I also liked our Black History Month displays.

We talked about the journeys taken by different groups of people through history and their contributions to society as a whole. I loved seeing students, visitors, and administrators notice and discuss our work. It was nice to see them linger for awhile on their way to lunch or class. I don't know if they were angry, annoyed, or just curious – whatever the reason, people noticed. We found a nonverbal way to make a powerful statement with those displays, and though I spent more time on them than I should have, I was proud that we found a way to reach out and get people talking about our message.

I really think that our entire medical school class was phenomenal, but nothing compared to SNMA. There were a handful of students intensely committed to community service, and we all wanted to give back in a big way. We worked really well together and fed off of each other to come up with some big ideas and the innovative programs. We had so much fun doing the work and can feel good about what we contributed to NJMS and its surrounding community.

Did you spend any time abroad during medical school or residency?

Luckily, yes. I like to travel and love international medicine. In medical school I wanted to do some travel to Africa. Two friends and I applied to a program focused on familiarizing students with health care delivery in third world areas. We were accepted and were all set up for a one-month trip to Cape Town, South Africa. We couldn't have been more excited! Unfortunately, a few days before we were supposed to leave, there were administrative issues with the program, so instead of going to Cape Town, we were rerouted to Mexico. Disappointment doesn't begin to describe how I felt when I found out, but somehow, it ended up being a good experience for me. I got to see how medicine is practiced in a place not as affluent as the United States. I got to see lots of gross pathology and observe surgeries performed with the bare minimum of tools and follow up care. The trip made me more appreciative of the modern conveniences that we have in our medical system. In residency, I was set up to do a mission trip where we would have spent 4-5 days doing gynecologic surgery and primary care in remote areas of Jamaica. Again, due to scheduling issues, my team and I couldn't go. I won't give up though - maybe next year we can go to Jamaica or Liberia. International medicine is definitely something I would like to incorporate into my practice after residency is all over.

The Application: Putting your best foot forward...

What was the most difficult part of the application/admission process for you?

Dealing with fear. Fear that my grades and board scores would void all of the hard work I did during medical school, and prevent me from moving forward in my career. I actually liked writing my personal statement and putting the whole application together – that part wasn't so difficult. As I went through it all though, making it as presentable and appealing as I could, the reality of getting into residency started to sink in. I had decided to pursue obstetrics and gynecology (OB-GYN), which at that time, was very popular. Lots of people were going into that field, and that introduced a lot of anxiety. I had dreamt big, and silently dealt with major concerns about how things would turn out for me.

Tell me about the people that helped with your application.

There were a bunch of people that helped. I used my dad a lot. He's a professor of clinical psychology, but used to be an English teacher. He has a great mastery of the English language, so I used him for creativity, editing, and proofreading. Many of the faculty members at my school also looked over my personal statement and made sure that I was properly highlighting the activities and awards that obstetric programs would look for. Our vice-dean looked over the section on work experience, and thanks to her help, I had all of the pertinent information in there. Our dean for student affairs also helped to incorporate personal things into my personal statement. The department of obstetrics was also wonderful – even our department's chairman sat with me and helped put the polish on my application before it went out.

Testing My Patience: The USMLE...

Tell us about your USMLE testing experiences.

My USMLE experience is still going on, and it is truly my Achilles heel. It was the bane of my existence during medical school and it almost defines me now; even though I know it shouldn't. I think I have always struggled with test taking to some degree, but definitely, the USMLE has been a big hurdle. My scores have always been just shy of the mark - with Step 1, I failed by 2 points, Step 2 was only 1 point. Step 3 was by a lot more, but still it's frustrating to work so hard and come so close, only to face another failure. My process for dealing with those tests is always the same - I get sad, cry my eyes out, feel like I'm dumb, and then I put it behind me. Before I get too down on myself, I remember that I've gotten so far and have accomplished a lot. I never think about giving up. My grandmother instilled a fighting spirit in me, and because of her, I will never quit. Sure, my experience has not been completely positive – and the USMLE is probably the most negative thing about my medical journey - but once the depression clears, I reach down somewhere inside and figure out what needs to happen in order to move forward.

Where did you go for help? What methods did you try while studying?

You name it – I've done it. Ever since college I've done one-on-one study sessions with professors, used flash cards, and employed various memorization techniques.

When I started medical school though, I realized that I was not studying properly. I would put lots of time in, but it wasn't high yield. I next figured out that I was a visual and oral studier, so I started doing group study, dry erase boards, and constant repetition. When I started having problems with Step 1, I even told my dad that I perhaps had a learning disability and needed to be evaluated for that. He assured me that a problem of that sort would have manifested itself a lot earlier in my schooling, so we were back to square one. We read books on test taking strategies and worked with specialists to figure the root problem. Unfortunately no one has been able to uncover the answer to that question, so I'm still just studying as much as possible and praying for a good outcome. If I were to count the vast number of hours I've spent studying, no one would believe it, especially if they were to compare it to my test scores. Something just goes into my head when I sit for these tests and causes me to either draw a blank, or doubt myself when it's time to come up with an answer. To deal with this, I have figured out how to make all of my studying high yield, making sure that I understand all of the material, can regurgitate the information, explain it in a simple way, and incorporate it into my work day. I have used formal programs like Kaplan and whatever structured courses that my school offered. Also important is to avoid being tired, distracted, or unfocused. I know that my optimal time for studying is morning or early afternoon, but definitely not late at night. In college, I observed a program that would teach kids to preserve their mind, body, and soul at all costs. They would do exercises, eat healthy foods, and channel into whatever spiritual avenues they chose. I have certainly tried to incorporate that, and though I'm not always successful, it really does give me the energy to deal with academic issues and life in general.

Do troubles with test taking translate into difficulties performing during residency itself?

The frustrating part is that it doesn't at all. I am a great physician, and take care of my patients very well. I can recall information in order to treat a certain ailment or perform a certain procedure, but just not to pass the necessary tests the first time around. The reality of the situation is that I need to pass Step 3 to get my medical license, my DEA number, and be a solo practitioner, so I guess I'll continue working to make that happen every time around...

Interview Trials: Finding the best fit...

Tell me about the interviews you went on.

Interviews were interesting. Some programs gave me interviews perhaps because they thought my personal statement was unique. I remember one interviewer being very impressed by the mention of articles I had written for our school newspaper. I didn't think it was a big deal – I had simply written about things that caught my attention. We talked at length about my article topics - genetically modified foods, clean water resources, and malaria – random things that I was interested in. The interviewers thought that it showed a different perspective and that I was a candidate not only passionate about medicine, but also reaching out and helping with broad public health concerns.

As I mentioned I was very worried about my USMLE test scores during the application process. I had to take both Step 1 and 2 twice, and was nervous that it would be the entire focus of all of my interviews. I came to all interviews prepared with a fool-proof strategy addressing that problem. I was ready to talk about a strength, a weakness, and any areas on my application that needed explaining. My three-part response to questions about weaknesses was to acknowledge the problem, list the steps I took to correct the situation, and end on a positive note – telling what I learned from the ordeal, and how I can use that knowledge to make me a better physician. So my Genetics course didn't go well, but I did x, y, and z to rectify things, and even started doing research in the field with my professor. This was a very mature approach to dealing with less than desirable grades or experiences. I never put blame on anyone else for my shortcomings. I took responsibility for the things that happened and helped interviewers see that if placed in a similar situation during residency, I would find a way to turn it around for the good of my patient and the program.

Surprisingly, only two interviewers discussed my scores and let me know that it was going to be an issue for them. For the most part, programs focused on my personal statement – the research I did, the organizations that I worked with, my future goals. Obviously all programs look at academics, but if you put information on your application showing them that you are a real person with lots to offer, you can't go wrong with that.

Any bad interview experiences?

There were definitely places that I knew weren't going to be for me. They were good programs, and they may be perfect for others, but when I walked in, everything about the hospital rubbed me the wrong way. One place felt almost like some sort of prison, and their attitude certainly didn't help things. I felt like I was part of a herd of cattle being moved in mass groups with no personal interaction. Usually programs try to introduce you to some residents so you get a sense of who you'd be working with and see how they handle the job. Here, we met a second year doctor that was so rude – she made no attempt to put a good face forward for the applicants or hide her contempt for the program. And as if that wasn't bad enough, the interviewers asked questions that were way too personal. They asked whether I was married, and if I planned to have children in the near future. These types of questions are illegal during interviews, but I guess they wanted to see if I would be willing to sacrifice family for work. Needless to say, I did not put this program on my rank list. I didn't want to risk having to go there for residency, and since you are not always guaranteed your top three rank choices, I played it safe and avoided what could have been a terrible situation.

When 24 Hours Isn't Enough...

Tell me about a typical day for you – preferably a call day if possible.

Now that I'm a senior resident and don't have as many patients to round on as I did as an intern or junior, I usually arrive around 6am. I arrive, see my assigned patients, write notes, then go to sign-out. Sign-out begins at 6:30am for us, and is where the entire team gets together to discuss patients. We talk about overnight events with the team that was on call the night before, and they tell us what to follow up on and what medical issues to keep an eye out for. That team goes home, then the rest of us talk about the remaining patients on our service. The juniors are in charge of the obstetric patients - anywhere from 5-30, depending on how busy things are. The seniors handle the management of gynecologic and high risk patients.

After sign-out, things can get crazy. On my last call day, there was lots of activity carrying over from the night before, so we had a very quick sign-out. I had to rush to the operating room to join the surgery on a woman who had developed a massive hematoma. Her blood levels (or hematocrit) were dangerously low, she had no urine output, and her blood pressure wouldn't stay up in a normal range. We opened her up in hopes of finding the source of her bleeding, and emptied almost a liter of blood from her belly in huge clots. Sometimes we never actually find the source of bleeding, and in this case, we spent two or three hours, and gave her multiple units of replacement blood.

When this surgery was over, I returned to the floor, and tried to help my junior prioritize patients and work

179

assignments. We had laboring women to check up on constantly, and had to see new patients in the emergency room. Plus, we had to deal with the complicated gyn-onc (cancer) patients on the floor. One woman had gotten a thermal burn injury on her uterer (the connection between the bladder and the outside world) after a previous surgery. She developed a severe infection and had to be taken back to the OR. During my entire call day, I kept checking on her to make sure that she was getting better. There is a lot of this that goes along with being on call. You manage any obstetric emergencies that come through the door, like cord prolapse or early labor. You handle difficult patients, demanding attendings, or unfavorable situations. In the times when things are slow, you can read or rest, interact with nurses, or most importantly, eat! Basically, you need to be ready at the drop of a dime and stay sharp as a tack. You need to be a team player, and just keep the best interests of the patients in mind.

When you are on call are you in the hospital by yourself?

For obstetrics and gynecology there is always an attending in house with us. If, for instance, we have to go to the OR suddenly with a bleeding ectopic pregnancy case, there wouldn't be enough time for an attending to drive to the hospital to save her. The patient could die very quickly during a long wait, so there is always an in-house attending, a senior and a junior in our program. Most of the time the attending is asleep and I check in with them if I need anything, but in emergencies, it's wonderful to have them around.

How overwhelming would you say your job is, if at all?

Hmmm – it has gotten better. Medical school was so great, and after Match Day, I was on a natural high. I was hanging with my family and friends, thinking 'I'm done', and 'I've accomplished this and that', etc. You really don't think about what's ahead for you. Then July hits, and you get your dreaded pager. You can't say 'Oh, I can't answer that question for you because I'm just a medical student', because guess what - you are the doctor! People are looking to you for answers and you better come up with something. I know that it can seem like too much. I felt like I didn't have time to do anything other than work when I first started. I was getting depressed for a long time, thinking 'I can't do this'. I held on to this defeated attitude, knowing that it wasn't helping my patients one bit.

Now that I'm a senior, I've had a lot of really bad days, so I've gotten comfortable with it. My first senior call was April 5, 2008 – I remember it clearly. The night before I was very nervous and couldn't sleep. I couldn't believe I was going to be the senior. What would I do if all the bad things that *could* happen while on call *did* happen? Could I fix things? Would my anxiety get in the way of doing a good job?   I had so much on my mind, and of course it ended up being the worst call ever – almost all the complications and emergencies that could happen did. There were some really critical patients; some had to go to the ICU.   A couple of babies had to be delivered by c-section in less than a minute because there was no audible heartbeat.   For one of them, I was alone with the nurses in the room, and didn't even wait for the attending to come in. I called it, got to the operating table, and had the baby out in 30 seconds!   It was a crazy day.   My favorite part, though, was when the next day came around.   I looked around and exclaimed, 'Wait – I'm still standing!'.   I survived, and for the most part we had good outcomes.   We did our best for the patients and kept them all stable.   My fears never materialized; ever since, I haven't felt as overwhelmed as I did on that long, long day.

I've learned to just take a deep breath and tackle the work.   Even if, in my mind, I feel overwhelmed, I never show it because that never helps any situation.   I have to be able to run the show, so if I'm not calm, no one else is going to be calm.   We've all seen the nervous attendings who throw everyone else off their game.   I decided that even if I'm not confident about what I'm doing, I'll process my fears and insecurities later – after the patient is safely recovering.   My field is definitely demanding, but you really have to hit the ground running, keep learning, and build your confidence every chance you get.   If you do that, you, too, will one day look around and be proud of the progress you've made, and the difference you've made in the lives of your patients.

Family Ties: Life outside of the OR...

Tell me how you manage your time between friends, family, work, relationships, church.

When I started residency I was in a relationship with someone. I thought that would be a positive thing for me, so I did everything possible to make time for the relationship and help it grow. Even if I had to drive all the way to South Jersey from Connecticut every Friday, then turn around to be back home in time for a 4am wake up call on Monday, it was important enough to me to do it. Studying, family time and church time had to fit in also, so I kept asking for more than 24 hours in the day. For some reason, God wouldn't give it to me, so I figured that I ought to just make the most of the hours I had to work with.

I have to do things for work – can't get around that. Church is a huge part of my life - that's what keeps me going. It rejuvenates me, and is important enough that even if I'm tired, I go. Unless I'm on night float or on call, I consult my church schedule to keep up with my meetings and events as much as possible. With my friends, I have a circle of good buddies that I also love spending time with, and I do a lot to keep those relationships going. I'm not a phone or letter person, so I try to see people, even if I have to travel to where they are. A group of us tries to get together at least once a year, and all vacations and free weekends are put to good use.

It's a hectic life trying to juggle all these things, but it's worth it. I have a friend from medical school who always took Friday evenings as her "me time". She would pick a time on Friday nights to pack her bags and head out, even if we were in the middle of studying. She had something to look forward to throughout the week, and would budget her time in order to fit in a little relaxation. It was important to her, and I would love to start doing that myself. I don't do a lot of "me time" – if I had to do it all over again I would factor that in because it helps keep you sane and believe it or not, more focused.

What has surprised/disappointed you about residency?

I never thought that I would hate patients. Honestly, I used to think that I would automatically love even the nastiest patients, but I've gotten to a point now where even the sight of some of them leaves a bad taste in my mouth. I really don't want to feel that way, but it is hard to put up with some of the folks that come through our doors. There are patients who take ambulances to the hospital just for a pregnancy test. There are women who refuse to take care of themselves regardless of our best medical advice. It's frustrating to go out of your way and never get through to some people.

I'll also never get over the fact that no one outside of medicine seems to know exactly what a resident is. Some don't think we're "real" doctors, even though we've graduated medical school, have a medical license, and have a degree hanging on our walls. No one knows what we do all day, or what it means to be on call. They think you're at home, sipping lattes, when you're actually doing the work that the entire team would be doing during normal working hours. No one gets why you're tired all the time, regardless of the fact that you just told them that you spent the last 30 hours running through a hospital in nonstop high-adrenaline situations. I used to think I could explain it once or twice to family and friends, but I get the same questions and blank stares all the time. Very frustrating.

The difficulty of dealing with hospital dynamics also surprised me when I came to residency. Between nurses expecting you to know everything, and attendings assuming that you know nothing – it's a weird feeling. Handling the family members of your patients can be the

184

most difficult thing of them all. I once was post-call, but instead of bolting out of the hospital, I decided to help the oncoming team since it was a busy day. I went to the emergency room just to inform a family that their sister had been taken to surgery. They immediately started yelling at me, wouldn't let me get two words in, and then started throwing insults around. I calmly stated, "I don't know what specifically is going on, but we will work it out." When more yelling started, I said "I've been up for the last 24 hours and it's been a very busy day." Instead of listening and being reasonable, they shot back, "We don't care about what you've been doing – it's your damn job." I'll never get used to behavior like that!

Next Steps...

What's next for you after residency?

Assuming that I pass Step 3 and my OB-GYN boards, I have decided that I don't want to do a fellowship for more training after residency. I could do more training in gynecologic oncology, maternal fetal medicine (perinatology), urogynecologic/pelvic surgery, or reproductive endocrinology/infertility. I have nothing but respect for those who choose fellowship, but I've known for awhile that it wasn't for me. I'm not interested in those things, so it would be a waste of time for me to pursue those areas. I chose a community program for that reason, since I knew I didn't want fellowship – but I also wanted a program affiliated with an academic institution just in case I changed my mind.

I would like to run a community clinic in my future. It's definitely not as lucrative as a big private office practice, but that's what I want. Even now, as a resident, I come alive in the clinic, and can truly say that I love all of my clinic patients. I have had lots of difficulties with them, but the clinic is where I do my best work. I get to take care of the whole person, unlike in the hospital, where you have to focus on the one or two issues that are jeopardizing their health. After starting off in a community clinic, I plan to lay the foundation for a Women's Health Clinic – possibly overseas. I've already lined up potential physician partners, now I just need funding and a great location.

I've always been drawn to doing things in the community - not that anyone *has* to. Some people will tell you that you owe something to your community, and that you must do certain things to give back. I say that you've worked hard to get to a certain position in life, so you don't need to explain yourself, or excuse the choices you've made for yourself. What drives *me* is giving back though. I'm a big proponent of helping young black females, because I can identify with them. I've had similar experiences to them, and so that's where I focus my attention. I'll see 15 year old patients who just delivered their second baby. They have terribly low self-esteem, and may have even experienced abusive relationships. After I go through the general medical questions & their annual exam, I always incorporate a talk about their goals and plans. I ask about their interests, and talk with them about self-empowerment

There is one girl at my hospital that works in food services and wants to be a doctor. Growing up, her guidance counselor told her that she wouldn't be able to cut it as a physician, she would be in debt, and she wouldn't be able to handle the work load. She and I would talk over Italian icees in the cafeteria, or during rides in the elevator. I tell her that she can do it, and that I'll need compassionate, caring people like her to take care of me when I'm old and out of the business. There's also a scrub technician that works in the operating room with me. She wants to be a family practice doctor, but thinks she has too many responsibilities to make it happen. I always push her to go for it, and now, she's taking classes at a local community college and is almost done with her basic science courses. I think it's so important to help others realize their potential and achieve the things in life that they really want. Where would any of us be without the support and guidance of those around us? I remember that when I interact with these patients and co-workers, and I know that I'll continue to do this throughout my career.

Any last minute thoughts?

Whatever you want to do as a student, you can do it. If medicine is what you really want, sure, applying to medical school or residency programs is hard, but you will do it and you will get in. Choose a field that really intrigues you, and don't let your own negative thinking get in the way. I didn't think I could do obstetrics because there's a lot of surgery involved, but now, I love it and am good at it. If you want to be a neurosurgeon, that's what you should do. Lots of people will challenge you – attendings, other residents, even yourself. Just remember that it's going to be hard work, but it will definitely be worth it! Surround yourself with loving, supportive people, and find a suitable outlet, whether it's music, exercise – whatever. You have to look beyond your present situation and never get too down about the hardships that you face. That's easy for me to say, since I can see the light at the end of the tunnel, but never, never give up, regardless of what happens. Remember why you are doing this; cry and get angry if you have to. But after everything, you must refocus, and figure out how you'll get to the next level. You can definitely do it!!!

CAREER SNAPSHOT

IN FOCUS: OBSTETRICS & GYNECOLOGY

Years in graduate school: 4 years medical school

Years in post-graduate training: 4 years residency

Fellowship: maternal/fetal medicine, reproductive endocrinology/infertility, etc.

Salary: average annual salary ranges from $230,000 to $300,000 and up

Pros: addresses women's health, can be practiced with surgical or medical focus

Cons: high liability/malpractice insurance required

Extra info: malpractice premiums can be as high as $100,000 per year in some areas!

Information taken from http://www.aamc.org/cim

"Been There, Done That"

What follows is an informative interview conducted by the *So You Wanna Be A Doctor* editors with two attending physicians who have a combined 60 years of experience as top-notch physicians under their belt. They interact with students, residents, and fellows daily and can tell you exactly what can guarantee success in medicine...

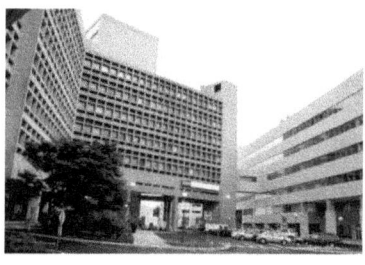

Trevor H. Atherley, M.D., P.A.
Cardiology
F.R.C.P. (c). F.A.C.C.

Leon S. Dick, M.D., P.A.
General Surgery
Vascular Surgery

SYWBAD: What does your job specifically entail? What do you do and what are you responsible for?

THA: Well there are multiple aspects of the job. In terms of my own private practice – I'm an interventional cardiologist – it involves seeing patients in a variety of clinical circumstances, cardiology consultations, admissions to the hospital, as well as doing certain procedures. I'm involved in invasive procedures like cardiac catheterizations and coronary angioplasty. The non-invasive procedures include echocardiograms and stress tests. So those are the work aspects, and there are administrative aspects to my job as well. I am the director of cardiac telemetry, where I am responsible for the day-to-day running of the telemetry units, or cardiac monitored units in the hospital. I help select residents to train in our fellowship program, and I also do a great deal of teaching for the cardiology fellows, medicine residents, and interns. For the past week, I had high school students, so even for people not yet in medicine but simply interested in the field at that early stage, I occasionally have them come and observe what we do in cardiology and medicine.

LSD: My job is to do everything! I do general surgery procedures like gall bladder or gallstone removal, hernia repair, bariatric (weight loss) surgery. I also do vascular surgery which includes dialysis graft creation and repair, varicose vein removal, and leg ulcer care. This is slightly atypical in this day and age because most surgeons stick to either vascular or general surgery, but I chose to do both. I have stayed away from many of the

190

endovascular procedures that carry high radiation exposure risks. There is documented hand, eye, and body exposure to and absorption of ionizing radiation during operations that involve fluoroscopy, and in my practice I choose not to do as many of those. I operate in a private practice setting. I have my own office, am in charge of my own staff, and also try to teach students as much as possible.

SYWBAD: Why do you like working with students and residents? Why is that an important thing to focus on?

LSD: Because eventually someone will have to take care of us in the older generation, and we want them to be the best they can be. If they can benefit from our experience now – learn from our mistakes and avoid them as they take care of patients - that's a win-win situation.

THA: I agree. We teach them so that they can do what we do and build upon our knowledge and expertise. I enjoy teaching as a whole, but I love the fact that it also keeps me on my toes. My interaction is mostly with doctors at the fellowship level, but I do have interns and residents as well. Teaching involves things like journal club, where new articles are presented and we discuss the latest literature in cardiology. The young cardiology fellows are exposed to a number of different teachers, and we indirectly benefit from their exposure to varying techniques and approaches in the procedure room. They attend a variety of conferences and come back to discuss the information with us, helping us to learn from them while teaching them our craft.

SYWBAD: What do you look for in applicants or people to work with? What qualities are most important to you?

THA: In applicants for the fellowship of Cardiology, we have a pretty broad pool to draw from. For example, in the selection process involved in our program, we see individuals who have completed their internships and are final year residents. We look at the programs that they are in, the medical schools they come from, and their recommendation letters from program directors and others. We go all the way back to basic scores for standardized examinations that they have taken over the years. We start off with hundreds and narrow that pool down to about 10 applicants to come for the actual interview. There is a diverse group of cardiologists interviewing them, and they then make the final decision. At the time that we meet them, they have already been highly pre-screened, so we can sit and talk intently with them. We note their responses - not only academic, but attitudinal. We want to see what their interests are and how strong their character is. It's a bit of a pressure situation for the applicants, for they come into a room filled with renowned cardiologists from all over the world and are understandably nervous. How they handle that situation tells us a lot about how they will handle their time in cardiology. We observe carefully then select based on their performance. After all is said and done, we are able to comfortably select from that broad initial pool 2 or sometimes 3 fellows to join us in the program.

LSD: The process in surgery is similar, except that today, I think it's more of a crapshoot. Decades ago, we applied to 2 or 3 programs and focused our energy on getting familiar with them in order to gain acceptance. Today, some applicants apply to as many as 50 different programs and just hope for the best. Those in charge of the programs have a difficult time choosing among hundreds of applications and finding the 3 or 4 residents that will be the best fit for their hospital and team.

SYWBAD: Speaking of the admissions process, when it comes to personal statements, should they be flowery and poetic, a boastful list of their every accomplishment, or an apologetic rant about the mistakes they've made in school?

LSD: They should be truthful and they should make mention of their accomplishments. It certainly should not be anything that is made up or exaggerated to attract attention. Statements like that tend to be transparent, and they don't tell the admissions committee member anything about the actual applicant.

THA: The ones that are genuine always look best. There are circumstances where we are influenced by life stories, for example people who have mentioned that they have been interested in my specialty from an early age because a parent had a severe heart problem. Also, it is refreshing to hear about some of the struggles and triumphs that people have gone through to reach the resident or fellow level. If it is well written and moving, these stories do influence us to some extent. We also want an explanation of some accomplishments and major interests. I must stress, however, that these things only go a small way in helping us make a selection. They may help choose between A and B, but by and large, it is the academic qualifications and the ability of the individual that seals the deal.

SYWBAD: How is the choice for a residency or fellowship program best approached? What should be top on an applicant's list when looking at a program?

THA: I think a program that suits the applicant's needs is important to find. For example, people who want to go into academic medicine may choose programs accordingly that will expose them to more research and didactics. People that want to go into more practical programs may look at the number of cases of X done at a particular place, and say 'that's what I'm looking for'. We do a lot of interventional studies and have one of the most active cath labs in the country at our program. An applicant would have to look at the statistics and decide if that is for them. Other things would have some weight also – location (urban? suburban?), the number of fellows or residents, how hard they'll have to work, how often they're on call, etc. Many, many things play a part, and I think they should be individualized based predominately on the person's lifestyle and what they want after they finish their program.

LSD: For general surgery, obviously it's very different than vascular surgery when coming out of medical school. General surgery means at least 5 years in residency after med school. Vascular surgery can be done as an integrated 5-year surgical program, or as a surgical residency plus vascular surgery fellowship. Once you've identified your specific specialty and your top choices, I advise calling the residents training there in order to get a flavor of what the program is really like. If you want to do academic surgery with teaching and research, then naturally, you would go to a program more attuned to academic pursuits. However, if you are more interested in seeing patients and performing in the operating room, it is easy to research how a particular program stacks up. There are many websites and books that can guide you, as well as advisors and current professionals with invaluable personal experiences. I cannot overstate the importance of visiting a program and visualizing yourself working and thriving there.

SYWBAD: What are the best resources for aspiring doctors?   Are there any books or websites that you routinely recommend to students?

THA: I don't know exactly what students do now-a-days, but you can never go wrong speaking to current residents or those who recently completed residency. They will tell you what helped them, and what kinds of things their hospital or program looks for.

SYWBAD: What have your years in medicine taught you?

LSD: It has taught me that 80% of what you read is useless. Sure, you need all of it to build a foundation, but medicine changes so rapidly that the things you read today may be obsolete in a few years. You need to be skeptical of much of what comes out. Luckily, every so often there are breakthroughs in knowledge that lead to improvements in outcomes and patient care. Those are the things that make a difference, and that is why remaining current with medical literature and continuing medical education is so important for us today.

THA: I suppose there have been a large number of lessons that my years have taught me. It has taught me the value of experience and confidence - borne out by experience and improved expertise. It taught me the importance of the patients themselves and not just the books. There are so many different lessons that one learns, but you come to realize that yes, you will learn a lot, and that continues long after you complete your basic fundamental training.

SYWBAD: Well thank you very much for your time, Doctors. This has been a wonderful interview experience, and we hope that our readers take some valuable lessons away from your chapter.

CAREER SNAPSHOT

IN FOCUS: CARDIOLOGY

Years in graduate school: 4 years medical school

Years in post-graduate training: 3 years Internal Medicine residency

Fellowship: clinical cardiac electrophysiology, interventional cardiology, etc.

Salary: average annual salary ranges from $250,000 to $400,000 and up

Pros: many hands-on procedures possible

Cons: possible long hours, must focus on lifestyle choices for patients

Extra info: there are 179 cardiovascular disease fellowships available in this country

Information taken from http://www.aamc.org/cim

CAREER SNAPSHOT

IN FOCUS: GENERAL SURGERY

Years in graduate school: 4 years medical school

Years in post-graduate training: 5 years residency

Fellowship: hand surgery, vascular surgery, pediatric surgery, etc.

Salary: average annual salary ranges from $270,000 to $350,000 and up

Pros: diagnose and definitively treat many conditions

Cons: high risk of further injury/illness with each surgical procedure

Extra info: surgeons provide increasing amount of care through minimally invasive and endoscopic techniques

Information taken from http://www.aamc.org/cim

CODE BLUE

20 Do's and Don'ts For Surviving An Emergency Situation

When you are the doctor on call and the code light goes off, what do you do? How do you react? What will help you through? Remember these simple tips and you'll be fine!

1. TAKE A DEEP BREATH

   Going into a life-or-death situation can be scary. Before you rush into the action, take a deep breath, slow things down, and collect yourself. That way, you'll be on top of your game!

2. KNOW YOUR SURROUNDINGS

   Where is this emergency taking place? Are you in a hospital where there is lots of equipment around, or are you in a shopping mall, school, or outdoor space where you'll have to be more resourceful?

3. GATHER LOTS OF INFORMATION

   What exactly is the emergency? Is someone choking? Has someone passed out? Who is having the emergency? Is the patient on medications? Did they just have surgery? The more you know, the better your decisions will be.

4. ACT QUICKLY

   Do a quick survey then start moving! Gather the tools needed and put a plan into action.

5. GET HELP

Involve nurses, technicians, other doctors – even family members. If you are not in a hospital setting, give clear instructions to those around you and get started!

6. BE SAFE AND STERILE
    Gloves are a must! If you are near a pair, put them on. Face shields and gowns couldn't hurt; also carefully remove the patient from any fire, deep water, or other threatening area.

7. PUT THE PATIENT FIRST
    Remember that this patient needs your help and is depending on you for their survival. Go the extra mile and give them the care they deserve.

8. DON'T GUESS – BE CERTAIN
    Do I give Atropine or Epinephrine first? Do I do the Heimlich maneuver or place the patient in recovery position? Know what you are doing, and don't forget to get help if you need it!

9. DELEGATE RESPONSIBILITY
    You cannot do it all and there are people around who can help. Let someone else start the IV. Take turns doing chest compressions. Remember it's all for the benefit of the patient!

10. REMAIN CALM
    Again, take a deep breath. Take things one step at a time. Everyone works better in a calm environment, and so will you!

11. BE SYSTEMATIC

If there are algorithms available, now is the time to remember them. BLS and ACLS protocols are there to assist you, so use them when necessary.

12. OBEY PATIENT WISHES

While gathering information, find out if this patient has a DNR order on the chart. If he/she does not wish to have CPR performed on them, find another way to solve their health problem.

13. DON'T DO HALF THE JOB

Just because you cannot perform CPR, don't just walk away and give up. If a patient has an obvious gunshot wound in the abdomen, don't forget to examine the back for more injuries. Take care of the *whole* patient and do all that you can!

14. REMEMBER YOUR SAFETY

Back injuries, falls, and electrocutions can occur if health care professionals are not careful when attending to their patients. Always be aware of what is happening around you.

15. THINK THINGS THROUGH

Does this patient have glaucoma? Well then you may want to rethink giving Atropine. Remember all co-existing diseases, allergies, and medications so that you don't miss anything.

16. INVOLVE THE ENTIRE TEAM

Don't leave medical students, nursing assistants, or any health professional sitting on the sidelines. Everyone can play a role during an emergency, so whether you provide some teaching points, or have them man the computer, there is a place for the whole team.

17. DON'T PANIC

As a medical professional, you have the training and knowledge necessary to carry you through an emergency. Rest assured on that fact.

18. BE THOROUGH

Check all systems and orifices in a trauma situation. Try different approaches. Think of all possible scenarios. Get help from different disciplines. Do all that you can!

19. DON'T GET DISTRACTED

Keep your focus on the patient on the table and the situation at hand. Please don't start thinking about tomorrow's surgery, or yesterday's test scores. Stay in the moment and devote all of your attention to what you are doing.

20. HAVE FAITH IN YOURSELF

You can do this. You have been working towards this for years, and you are smart enough to figure out the best approach in any situation. Don't second guess yourself – *you can do this*!!

ESSENTIAL RESIDENCY RESOURCES

Now that you have read the resident stories contained in this book, it's time to put it all together. What did you gather from your reading? Do you have a better sense of what happens after medical school? How about what it takes to get into and through a residency program? Let's take a look back at some themes and words of advice from our experienced contributors...

■■

Medicine is a difficult field that requires a lot of hard work in order to be successful. It may take a long time to reach your goal, and you may experience a few disappointments, but our contributors think it's definitely worth it!

You must be honest with yourself before you get into medicine. Do you have the stomach for it? The patience and integrity? How about the determination and resourcefulness? You've already picked up this book, so you may be on the right track!

There are numerous avenues available for help in medicine. Parents, family members, neighbors, friends, teachers, counselors, academic advisors and your personal physician are excellent resources for information and guidance. Don't be afraid to ask and don't wait too long before you seek help if you need it!

Explore, explore, explore! You may have an idea of what you want to do in medicine, but you will never know if that's the right fit for you until you try it out. Do summer programs, research, volunteer work, shadowing opportunities, and rotations in as many fields as possible. Even if it doesn't change your mind regarding specialty, at least you'll learn something new and have some fun.

- Think carefully about your planned specialty

- Select a helpful advisor – one that is experienced and capable

- Do your research: use career fairs, websites, and books

- Figure which courses are required for grad school acceptance

- Seek full exposure to as many specialties as you can

- Get help with your application and its presentation

- Start everything early in terms of applications

- Proofread your application and dig deep for personal statement

- Become familiar with the different match systems out there

- Know all deadlines & document requirements in advance

- Be prepared for a lot of trial and error; be flexible and honest

- Look closely at each of the programs to which you will apply – can you live in a particular city for 3-8 years? How is the climate? Can you get along with the people? Is there the opportunity to do research? What will your schedule be?

As we have seen from *So You Wanna Be A Doctor*, medicine is a wonderfully exciting field! There are many opportunities and many paths to success. That success can be yours – especially with the right support and thorough preparation. We have put together a list of books, websites, and organizations that will help along the journey to an M.D.,

D.O., D.D.S., D.M.D., or D.V.M.. Explore the lists that follow and take advantage of every resource available! And don't forget to contact your school's education office for even more information!

BOOKS

Taking My Place in Medicine: A Guide for Minority Medical Students; Sage Publications. C. Webb, 2000.

This book is designed to help minority students thrive personally and academically in medical school, to make a realistic assessment of their strengths and weaknesses, to successfully confront societal myths and stereotypes and to develop healthy strategies to meet academic, personal, and relationship needs.

Getting into a Residency: A Guide for Medical Students; K. Iserson; 5th Ed., 2000.

A step-by-step guide through the process of selecting a medical specialty and obtaining a residency position. A unique 500 page book providing invaluable and practical information about all the medical specialties.

First Aid for the Match: Inside Advice from Students and Residency Directors; T. Le, V. Bhushan, 4th Ed., 2006.

Helps you to fully understand the match process, and increase your chances of getting in. Gives hints on writing a personal statement and curriculum vitae, and includes great advice on successfully navigating interviews.

Medical Student Guide to Successful Residency Matching 2000-2001; L. Miller.

Annual pocket guide to the year-long residency matching process. Covers specialty selections, planning clinical years, the matching process, selecting programs for application, interviewing, ranking, match day, and tips for the international medical graduate. Includes an appendix of resources.

Graduate Medical Education Directory (Green Book); AMA; 2001 Ed.

Newly revised by the AMA, the *Graduate Medical Education Directory, 2007 - 2008* (or the "Green Book") contains extensive information on more than 8,300 residency, fellowship and combined programs in the United States, as well as residency application and career-planning resources to help in making one of the most important professional decisions that a medical student can make.

101 Tips to Getting the Residency You Want: A Guide for Medical Students; J. Canaday

Guiding residency applicants past the pitfalls in all aspects of the process, this book includes sections on tried-and-true methods for senior year planning, the importance of networking, tips for interviewing, practical advice for carefree travel, and guidelines for follow-up to out-of-town rotations and interviews.

So You Want to Be a Brain Surgeon? A Medical Careers Guide; (2nd edition) Editors: Chris Ward, Simon Eccles; Oxford: Oxford Univ Press, 2001

Personal testimonies from experienced practitioners in more than 90 medical specialties. Focuses on medical education and practice in the U.K., but is also an excellent resource for medical students and newly minted doctors in the U.S.

INTERNET

National Resident Matching Program (NRMP) :
http://nrmp.aamc.org/nrmp/

Official site for everyone participating in the Main Match. The NRMP is a non-profit program that works to match applicants with appropriate positions in dozens of medical specialties.

San Francisco Matching Program :
http://www.sfmatch.org/

Official site for early match specialties and fellowships. Coordinates the processing, distribution and review of applicants for post graduate medical education training programs in Ophthalmology, Plastic Surgery, Child Neurology/Neurodevelopmental Disabilities, Neurotology, and their associated fellowships.

American Urological Association (AUA) Residency Match : *http://www. auanet.org*

Official site for urology residency match. Your one-stop for all information related to urology, including programs, deadlines, meetings, and resources.

Electronic Residency Application Service (ERAS) : *http://www.aamc.org/students/eras*

The Electronic Residency Application Service if a fee-for-service company that "transmits residency applications, letters of recommendation, Dean's Letters/MSPE, transcripts, and other supporting credentials from applicants and medical schools to residency programs.

Fellowship & Residency Electronic Interactive Database Access *: www.ama-assn.org/go/freida*

FREIDA Online is a database with over 8,600 graduate medical education programs accredited by the Accreditation Council for Graduate Medical Education, as well as over 200 combined specialty programs. Search for programs by specialty, state, institution, and optional criteria.

Internship & Residency Information Site (I-R-I-S) :
http://www.i-r-i-s.com/

> This site lists thousands of U.S. Internships
> & Residencies in all medical & surgical
> specialties, many with online program
> information and website links.

Accreditation Council for Graduate Medical Education
(ACGME) : *http://www.acgme.org/*

> The Accreditation Council for Graduate
> Medical Education (ACGME) is responsible for
> the accreditation of post-MD medical training
> programs within the United States.
> Accreditation is accomplished through a peer
> review process and is based upon
> established standards and guidelines.

World Directory of Medical Schools :
http://www.who.int/hrh/wdms/en/

> The WHO Department of Human Resources
> for Health, in collaboration with its partners,
> has been compiling information on education
> and training institutions for health workers
> around the world.

US News and World Report : *http://www.usnews.com*

> Medical School Rankings based on data from
> thousands of sources. These rankings allow
> students to narrow school search by location,
> tuition, size, and test scores. Also, find the

best schools in specialties such as pediatrics or rural medicine.

The Student Doctor Network :
http://www.Studentdoctor.net

A non-profit educational community for students and doctors spanning all the health care fields and specialties. Join talks on current medical concerns and get information on the application process.

Strolling Through the Match: A Medical Student's Guide :
Aafp.org/x20259.html

A guide for those seeking residency; helps the user get through NRMP and ERAS successfully.

CareerMD.com

Informational site for residency and beyond; a centralized source of knowledge on physician training and employment opportunities.

Medschool.com

General information to help you transition into residency and out of medical school.

Scutwork.com

A medical residency directory with ratings and reviews by people who have been there. Check out program reviews based on interviews and actual interactions.

Residentweb.com

Covers many topics of interest to residents (e.g., interviewing, student loans); includes forums where residents can share experiences.

Association of American Veterinary Medical Colleges :
http://www.aavmc.org

Up-to-date information on veterinary schools, conferences, training programs, and other resources.

American Dental Association : http://www.ada.org

Invaluable information on all things dental. Learn about the latest procedures and advances, related organizations, and dental schools.

MEDICAL ASSOCIATIONS

The **Association of American Medical Colleges** (AAMC) will act to meet its mission and fulfill its vision through the following nine strategic priorities:

- Serve as the voice and advocate for academic medicine on medical education, research, and health care
- Lead innovation along the continuum of medical education to meet the health needs of the public
- Facilitate development of a health system that meets the needs of all for access, safety, and quality of care
- Strengthen the national commitment to discovery that promotes health and enhances the treatment of disease and disability
- Lead efforts to increase diversity in medicine
- Be a valued and reliable resource for data, information, and services
- Help our members identify, implement, and sustain organizational performance improvement
- Provide outstanding leadership and professional development to meet the most critical needs of our members
- Nurture a culture at the AAMC that promotes excellence in service to our members and the public good

The **American Dental Education Association** (ADEA) is the voice of dental education. Its members include all U.S. and Canadian dental schools and many allied and postdoctoral dental education programs, corporations, faculty, and students. The mission of ADEA is to lead individuals and institutions of the dental education community to address contemporary issues influencing education, research, and the delivery of oral health care for the health of the public. ADEA's activities encompass a wide range of research, advocacy, faculty development, meetings, and communications like the esteemed *Journal of Dental Education,* as well as the dental school admissions services AADSAS and PASS.

The **Association of American Veterinary Medical Colleges** (AAVMC) represents all 32 veterinary medical colleges in the United States and Canada, nine departments of veterinary science, seven departments of comparative medicine, three veterinary medical education institutions, and six international colleges of veterinary medicine in its collective dealings with governmental bodies, veterinary medical organizations, the animal and human health industry, educational and scientific organizations and the public.

- American Medical Association
- American Dental Association
- Association of American Medical Colleges
- American Board of Medical Specialties
- American Medical Women's Association
- Council of Medical Specialty Societies
- Student National Medical Association
- Boricua Latino Health Organization
- American Veterinary Medical Association
- Asian Pacific American Medical Student Association

United States Medical Schools and Colleges

1. Albany Medical College (NY)
2. Albert Einstein College of Medicine of Yeshiva University (NY)
3. American Sports Medicine Institute (AL)
4. Boston University School of Medicine (MA)
5. Brown Medical School (RI)
6. Case Western Reserve University School of Medicine (OH)
7. Columbia University College of Physicians and Surgeons (NY)
8. Creighton University School of Medicine (NE)
9. Dartmouth Medical School (NH)
10. David Geffen School of Medicine, UCLA (CA)
11. Drexel University College of Medicine (PA)
12. Duke University School of Medicine (NC)
13. East Tennessee State Univ James H. Quillen College of Medicine (TN)
14. Eastern Virginia Medical School, Medical College of Hampton Roads (VA)
15. Emory University School of Medicine (GA)
16. Finch University of Health Sciences / The Chicago Medical School (IL)
17. George Washington University School of Medicine & Health Sciences (DC)
18. Georgetown University School of Medicine (DC)

19. Harvard Medical School (MA)
20. Howard University College of Medicine (DC)
21. Indiana University School of Medicine (IN)
22. Jefferson Medical College of Thomas Jefferson University (PA)
23. Joan & Sanford I. Weill Medical College of Cornell University (NY)
24. Joan C. Edwards School of Medicine at Marshall University (WV)
25. Johns Hopkins University School of Medicine (MD)
26. Keck School of Medicine of the University of Southern California (CA)
27. Loma Linda University School of Medicine (CA)
28. Louisiana State University School of Medicine in New Orleans (LA)
29. Louisiana State University School of Medicine in Shreveport (LA)
30. Loyola University Chicago Stritch School of Medicine (IL)
31. Mayo Medical School (MN)
32. Medical College of Georgia School of Medicine (GA)
33. Medical University of South Carolina College of Medicine (SC)
34. Meharry Medical College School of Medicine (TN)
35. Mercer University School of Medicine (GA)
36. Michigan State University College of Human Medicine (MI)
37. Morehouse School of Medicine (GA)
38. Mount Sinai School of Medicine of New York University (NY)

39. New York University School of Medicine (NY)
40. Northwestern University Medical School (IL)
41. Ohio State University College of Medicine and Public Health (OH)
42. Ponce School of Medicine (PR)
43. Rush Medical College of Rush University (IL)
44. Saint Louis University School of Medicine (MO)
45. Southern Illinois University School of Medicine (IL)
46. Stanford University School of Medicine (CA)
47. State Univ System - Downstate Medical Center College of Medicine (NY)
48. State University of New York System - Upstate Medical University (NY)
49. Stony Brook University Health Sciences Center School of Medicine (NY)
50. Temple University School of Medicine (PA)
51. The Brody School of Medicine at East Carolina University (NC)
52. Texas A&M Univ System Health Science Center College of Medicine (TX)
53. Tufts University School of Medicine (MA)
54. Tulane University School of Medicine (LA)
55. Uniformed Services University of Health Sciences – F. Edward Hebert School of Medicine (MD)
56. Universidad Central del Caribe School of Medicine (PR)

57. Buffalo State Univ of NY School of Medicine & Biomedical Sciences (NY)

58. University of Alabama School of Medicine (AL)

59. University of Arizona College of Medicine (AZ)

60. University of Arkansas College of Medicine (AR)

61. University of California Davis - School of Medicine (CA)

62. University of California Irvine - College of Medicine (CA)

63. University of California San Diego - School of Medicine (CA)

64. University of California San Francisco - School of Medicine (CA)

65. Univ of Chicago Division of Biological Sciences, Pritzker School of Med (IL)

66. University of Cincinnati College of Medicine (OH)

67. University of Colorado Health Sciences Center School of Medicine (CO)

68. University of Connecticut School of Medicine (CT)

69. University of Florida College of Medicine (FL)

70. University of Hawaii John A. Burns School of Medicine (HI)

71. University of Illinois College of Medicine (IL)

72. University of Iowa Roy J. and Lucille A. Carver College of Medicine (IA)

73. University of Kansas School of Medicine (KS)

74. University of Kentucky College of Medicine (KY)

75. University of Louisville School of Medicine (KY)
76. University of Maryland School of Medicine (MD)
77. University of Massachusetts Medical School (MA)
78. University of Medicine and Dentistry NJ - New Jersey Medical School (NJ)
79. Univ of Medicine and Dentistry NJ - Robert Wood Johnson Med School (NJ)
80. University of Miami School of Medicine (FL)
81. University of Michigan Medical School (MI)
82. University of Minnesota - Duluth School of Medicine (MN)
83. University of Minnesota Medical School - Twin Cities (MN)
84. University of Mississippi School of Medicine (MS)
85. University of Missouri-Columbia School of Medicine (MO)
86. University of Missouri-Kansas City School of Medicine (MO)
87. University of Nebraska College of Medicine (NE)
88. University of Nevada School of Medicine (NV)
89. University of New Mexico School of Medicine (NM)
90. University of North Carolina at Chapel Hill School of Medicine (NC)
91. University of North Dakota School of Medicine and Health Sciences (ND)
92. University of Oklahoma College of Medicine (OK)

93. University of Pennsylvania Health System (PA)
94. University of Pittsburgh School of Medicine (PA)
95. University of Rochester School of Medicine and Dentistry (NY)
96. University of South Carolina School of Medicine (SC)
97. University of South Dakota School of Medicine (SD)
98. University of South Florida College of Medicine (FL)
99. University of Tennessee Health Science Center College of Medicine (TN)
100. University of Texas Medical Branch at Galveston (TX)
101. University of Texas Medical School at Houston (TX)
102. University of Texas Medical School at San Antonio (TX)
103. University of Texas Southwestern Medical Center at Dallas Southwestern Medical School (TX)
104. University of Utah School of Medicine (UT)
105. University of Vermont College of Medicine (VT)
106. University of Virginia School of Medicine (VA)
107. University of Washington School of Medicine (WA)
108. University of Wisconsin Medical School (WI)
109. Vanderbilt University School of Medicine (TN)

110. Virginia Commonwealth University School of Medicine (VA)
111. Wake Forest University School of Medicine (NC)
112. Washington University in St. Louis School of Medicine (MO)
113. Wayne State University School of Medicine (MI)
114. West Virginia University School of Medicine (WV)
115. Wright State University School of Medicine (OH)
116. Yale University School of Medicine (CT)

United States Dental Schools and Colleges

Alabama: University of Alabama School of Dentistry

California: Loma Linda University School of Dentistry, University of California Los Angeles School of Dentistry, University of California San Francisco School of Dentistry, University of Southern California School of Dentistry. University of the Pacific School of Dentistry

Colorado: University of Colorado School of Dentistry

Connecticut: The University of Connecticut School of Dental Medicine

Florida: University of Florida College of Dentistry

Georgia: Medical College of Georgia School of Dentistry

Illinois: University of Illinois School of Dentistry

Indiana: Indiana University School of Dentistry

Kentucky: University of Kentucky School of Dentistry, University of Louisville School of Dentistry

Massachusetts: Boston University School of Dental Medicine, Harvard School of Dental Medicine, Tufts University School of Dental Medicine

Minnesota: University of Minnesota School of Dentistry

Mississippi: University of Mississippi School of Dentistry

Nebraska: Crieghton University School of Dentistry, University of Nebraska Medical Center

New Jersey: University of Medicine and Dentistry of New Jersey

New York: Columbia Presbyterian Medical Center School of Dental and Oral Surgery, New York University College of Dentistry, School of Dental Medicine - SUNY at Stony Brook, University at Buffalo School of Dentistry, University of Rochester School of Medicine & Dentistry

North Carolina: The University of North Carolina at Chapel Hill, School of Dentistry

Ohio: Case Western Reserve University School of Dentistry, Ohio State University School of Dentistry

Oklahoma: University of Oklahoma School of Dentistry

Pennsylvania: University of Pennsylvania School of Dentistry

South Carolina: Medical University of South Carolina

Tennessee: Meharry College of Dentistry

Texas: Baylor College of Dentistry, University of Texas Health Science Center at San Antonio, University of Texas - Houston Dental Branch

Washington: University of Washington School of Dentistry

Washington D.C.: Howard University

West Virginia: West Virginia University School of Dentistry

United States Veterinary Medical Schools and Colleges

Auburn University
Colorado State University
Cornell University
Iowa State University
Kansas State University
Louisiana State University
Michigan State University
Mississippi State University
North Carolina State University
Ohio State University
Oklahoma State University
Oregon State University
Purdue University
Texas A&M University
Tufts University
Tuskegee University
University of California, Davis
University of Florida
University of Georgia
University of Illinois at Urbana-Champaign
University of Minnesota
University of Missouri
University of Pennsylvania
University of Tennessee
University of Wisconsin-Madison
Virginia-Maryland Regional College of
Veterinary Medicine
Washington State University
Western University of Health Sciences

Canadian Veterinary Medical Schools and Colleges

Université de Montréal
University of Calgary
University of Guelph
University of Prince Edward Island
University of Saskatchewan

International Veterinary Medical Schools and Colleges

Massey University
Murdoch University
University College Dublin
University of Edinburgh
University of Glasgow
University of London
University of Melbourne
University of Sydney

Thank you for purchasing and reading

So You Wanna Be A Doctor??

The Untold Stories of Medical, Dental, and Veterinary Residents

Check us out on WagnerWolf.com for more exciting book titles, projects, and useful information!

Contact us whenever at wagnerwolfpublishing@yahoo.com Give us your feedback. Let us know what questions you still have!

See you in the health professions field!!

ABOUT THE AUTHORS

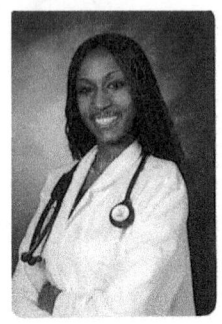

Wagner Wolf, LLC is headed by Shermian Daniel, M.D., our president. She is a resident physician in anesthesia, who is passionate about raising awareness of health issues like Multiple Sclerosis, Leukemias, and Obesity. She enjoys putting her writing skills to good use, and wishes to use this publishing company to reach students and involve them in community awareness.

ABOUT THE AUTHORS

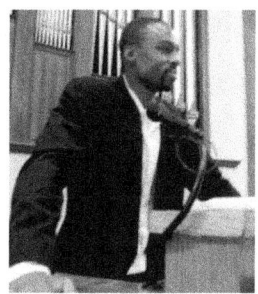

Wagner Wolf, LLC was co-founded by Richard Daniel, our vice-president. With a background in business, education, and multi-media production, he felt that establishing a publishing company would be the best way to incorporate all three fields and make a difference in the lives of those around him.

www.WagnerWolf.com